Feedback from Self-Practice/Self-Reflection

"Before SP/SR, I had an intellectual understanding of CBT, now I really know what it feels like! I am a therapist of many years' experience, but after doing SP/SR I have a very different and deeper understanding of the CBT approach than at any point in my career. I now see CBT through different eyes and practice it with a different level of compassion. Having been through this experience, I now believe strongly that every trainee and experienced therapist needs to do SP/SR. I now truly appreciate the level of honesty and effort required in the completion of apparently simple tasks like setting goals or completing questionnaires."

—SP/SR participant, Ireland

"I found SP/SR very useful. It was the first time I have had to complete a course that has had such a 'hands-on' part of the training. It was a great change to develop insight into my own processes and make the time to consider how and why I was feeling the way I was. This training component also cemented the theory we were reading and learning, and provided me with an insight into how the clients feel when asked to engage in cognitive therapy. I feel I shall be more enthusiastic in introducing the model into therapy than I initially was when I started. I shall be more enthusiastic when addressing the importance of homework completion."

—SP/SR participant, Australia

"[SP/SR was] . . . very useful—challenging to go through CBT interventions for oneself. Increases understanding and empathy for the clients and their work, and increased insights into my personal beliefs and related behaviors and how these limit my life; introduces the possibility of challenging and changing these."

—SP/SR participant, New Zealand

"SP/SR is a really powerful tool! It helped me to move away from ideas of inadequacy, which I had held on to and believed to be real for many years. I was doing SP/SR for the sake of it and I never expected it to affect me the way it did, both professionally and personally."

—SP/SR participant, Ireland

"What have I learned? . . . I thought I knew a lot about CBT, but looking back now, I only knew the surface of the iceberg (so to speak). This subject is a wonderful introduction into cognitive therapy . . . not only has it been useful to me in terms of my work, but also in my personal life. I have learned and been able to identify my strengths and weaknesses and come to terms with who I am and where I want to go in life."

—SP/SR participant, Australia

"Even now while reviewing this process I have had aha moments! I've decided it's OK to be more true to yourself. Hiding vulnerabilities doesn't really get you far. I can recognize when I've done this both at home and at work. For example, playing down that I don't want to progress in my career so I never have to try. Or playing down how much I want a family . . . I can laugh at this now. But my aha moments have been emotional ones at times. Not so much because of work stuff but recognizing how it has held me back in my personal life in the past."

—SP/SR participant, England

"I found the SP/SR component of the course really useful. I started off (as you may remember!!) very skeptical and suspicious, wondering where this level of analysis fit within an academic course. My reservations were not about the value of this sort of 'discovery' and self-awareness for us as clinicians and as people, just where this fit in the curriculum. . . . Just as SP/SR was essential for some professional insights about CBT unobtainable by other methods, similarly I had to experience the process of SP/SR in order to know its value."

—SP/SR participant, Australia

"I have to say that I have gained such a lot of insight into what it might feel like from the clients' perspective when they pitch up for help and that this experiential process has helped me to change lots of small things about the way I interact with clients, how I explain things, and the compassion I feel."

—SP/SR participant, England

"Both self-practice and self-reflection were the pivotal components of the course. Without them, it would have been impossible to achieve the level of understanding that comes from applying the material in a meaningful and critical way. For me personally, it was a chance of self-discovery that unearthed some amazing facets about the way I deal with my problems, as well as a true test of the cognitive-behavioral methods of intervention."

—SP/SR participant, Australia

"I have always related to CBT—it made sense to me so I really wanted to work with it. However, SP and SR have shown me what parts of my understanding were more at a surface level. SP/SR . . . greatly increased my understanding of how the techniques used are experienced by clients (particularly someone with no concept even of what CBT involves) and perhaps how these techniques work, not just a rational explanation of 'why' they work."

—SP/SR participant, Australia

"I think it was extremely valuable, both personally and professionally. I don't know how you can practice if you have not experienced what it is like yourself, how you can have any understanding or be able to anticipate what people are going to go through or what their own resistances and dilemmas might be, if you're not prepared to do that yourself."

—SP/SR participant, Australia

EXPERIENCING CBT FROM THE INSIDE OUT

SELF-PRACTICE/SELF-REFLECTION GUIDES FOR PSYCHOTHERAPISTS

James Bennett-Levy, Series Editor

This series invites therapists to enhance their effectiveness "from the inside out" using self-practice/self-reflection (SP/SR). Books in the series lead therapists through a structured three-stage process of focusing on a personal or professional issue they want to change, practicing therapeutic techniques on themselves (self-practice), and reflecting on the experience (self-reflection). Research supports the unique benefits of SP/SR for providing insights and skills not readily available through more conventional training procedures. The approach is suitable for therapists at all levels of experience, from trainees to experienced supervisors. Series volumes have a large-size format for ease of use and feature reproducible worksheets and forms that purchasers can download and print. Initial releases cover cognitive-behavioral therapy and schema therapy; future titles will cover acceptance and commitment therapy and other evidence-based treatments.

Experiencing CBT from the Inside Out:
A Self-Practice/Self-Reflection Workbook for Therapists
James Bennett-Levy, Richard Thwaites, Beverly Haarhoff,
and Helen Perry

Experiencing CBT from the Inside Out

A Self-Practice/Self-Reflection Workbook for Therapists

James Bennett-Levy
Richard Thwaites
Beverly Haarhoff
Helen Perry

Foreword by Christine A. Padesky

THE GUILFORD PRESS
New York   London

© 2015 The Guilford Press
A Division of Guilford Publications, Inc.
370 Seventh Avenue, Suite 1200, New York, NY 10001
www.guilford.com

Printed in the United States of America

This book is printed on acid-free paper.

Last digit is print number: 9   8   7   6   5   4   3   2   1

The authors have checked with sources believed to be reliable in their efforts to provide information
that is complete and generally in accord with the standards of practice that are accepted at the time of
publication. However, in view of the possibility of human error or changes in behavioral, mental health,
or medical sciences, neither the authors, nor the editors and publisher, nor any other party who has been
involved in the preparation or publication of this work warrants that the information contained herein
is in every respect accurate or complete, and they are not responsible for any errors or omissions or the
results obtained from the use of such information. Readers are encouraged to confirm the information
contained in this book with other sources.

Library of Congress Cataloging-in-Publication Data is available from the publisher

ISBN 978-1-4625-1889-0

To Concord—Ann, Melanie, Gillian, and Martina—
whose clinical skills and friendship
made my years at Oxford Cognitive Therapy Centre the richest of times
—JB-L

To Sarah for her encouragement and understanding,
and to all the staff within First Step
who have supported SP/SR and been part of a joint process of learning
—RT

To Errol, best friend and fellow traveler,
and to all the Massey University CBT postgraduate diploma students,
who have taught me so much
—BH

To my parents, whose pride in me never wavered,
and to Dave for the support and space provided,
especially through this journey
—HP

About the Authors

James Bennett-Levy, PhD, is Associate Professor in Mental Health at the University Centre for Rural Health, University of Sydney, Australia. He has pioneered self-experiential cognitive-behavioral therapy (CBT) training since his first self-practice/self-reflection (SP/SR) paper in 2001, and has made a significant contribution to the therapist training literature with over 25 CBT training publications. In particular, his 2006 Declarative–Procedural–Reflective model of therapist skill development is widely used and cited. Dr. Bennett-Levy is coauthor or coeditor of three other books on CBT practice, including, most recently, the *Oxford Guide to Imagery in Cognitive Therapy*.

Richard Thwaites, DClinPsy, is a consultant clinical psychologist and CBT therapist who serves as Clinical Director for a large National Health Service psychological therapies service in the United Kingdom. In addition to delivering therapy, he provides clinical leadership, supervision, training, and consultancy in CBT, including the implementation of SP/SR programs. His recent research interests include the role of the therapeutic relationship in CBT and the use of reflective practice in the process of skill development.

Beverly Haarhoff, PhD, is a clinical psychologist and Senior Lecturer in the School of Psychology at Massey University, Auckland, New Zealand, where she was instrumental in setting up the first Postgraduate Diploma in CBT in the southern hemisphere. For the past 14 years she has trained and supervised both CBT and clinical psychology trainees. Her research has focused primarily on SP/SR as mechanisms to support and improve therapist skill acquisition in CBT therapists at all levels of development. Dr. Haarhoff has a private clinical practice and regularly presents CBT training workshops.

Helen Perry, MA, is Adjunct Senior Lecturer at the University of Sydney and a clinical psychologist in private practice. She played a key role in creating the CBT Diploma Program at Massey University and is an active CBT trainer and supervisor. She served as Project Manager for a research study focusing on online CBT training and coauthored two papers in this area. Ms. Perry has worked across the lifespan in a wide range of clinical settings. Her special interests are in complex/comorbid depression and anxiety, and trauma- and stress-related disorders.

Foreword

One of the best ways to learn cognitive-behavioral therapy (CBT) is to use it in your own life. Only through weekly and daily practice do you appreciate the power of the methods used; their emotional, cognitive, and behavioral impact; and the obstacles that clients are likely to face when using them. For this reason, I was my first CBT client and have always included self-practice in my training programs and workshops.

What have I learned from my own self-practice of CBT and self-reflection? In addition to enjoying better moods and self-understanding, I've learned that my self-practice makes CBT more believable for my clients. Clients are often startled or moved when I say, "At first when I used this method, I found it difficult and yet after a few weeks it really helped me." Your credibility, the therapeutic alliance, and client adherence are enhanced when you have "walked the talk." Your personal experience using CBT speaks volumes to clients about your conviction that these methods are worthwhile.

I follow a personal rule to never give clients a homework assignment I have not either already done myself or which I plan to do in the coming week. Occasionally I say to clients, "Let's both do this assignment this week and compare notes on what happened when we see each other next session." Putting yourself through the same paces you expect of your client is a strong statement of your commitment to collaboration in therapy. It also serves as a reality check so you don't lose perspective on what it is like to do various learning tasks. And it emphasizes the importance of therapy experiments and learning exercises when you can say to the client, "I spend my time doing this as well."

Even a fundamental task such as identifying your automatic thoughts becomes richer when you take your time and attach quiet reflection to it. When I am feeling pressure at work and take a moment to notice my automatic thoughts, the first layer may be something akin to "I have so much to do. I must get this done today and there is barely time to do it." After identifying these initial automatic thoughts, I still feel pressured. However, if I spend more time attending to my thoughts, another layer emerges: "Others are counting on me. I want to do a good job." With a bit more reflective time, deeper levels of meaning come into focus: "It is really important to me that I do my best. I value this work and want to contribute. This is an opportunity for me to make a difference." When I take the time to uncover my automatic thoughts linked to deeper meanings and values, the pressure I feel may transform into an energized sense of purpose. Thus, if you want to learn how to use CBT most effectively, it is important you learn to practice it in ways that connect to deeper levels of awareness, not simply to superficial thoughts, emotions, and behaviors.

These concepts of self-practice are much better understood today than they were in the 1970s when I first learned to use CBT with myself and clients. I was delighted in 2001 when I was invited to be an examiner for James Bennett-Levy's doctoral dissertation, which was the first study of the effects of self-practice/self-reflection (SP/SR) on learning CBT. Bennett-Levy's idea of adding explicit self-reflection to self-practice was an important addition to the idea of learning by doing. The power of pairing practice and reflection has been borne out by research we later undertook together (Bennett-Levy & Padesky, 2014) and a number of SP/SR research studies conducted by the authors of this book. You will understand the concept of "from the inside out" by the time you finish this book.

As a reader, you are in good hands. The authors not only have used these methods themselves, they have guided hundreds of therapists through the process. The exercises, worksheets, and instructive text are all road-tested and designed to help you have the best experience possible using CBT for self-practice. The self-reflection exercises integrated into this book help you maximize your learning every step of the way. I'm pleased to see the emphasis in this book on identifying strengths, building new assumptions and behaviors, and the use of imagery and behavioral experiments. All these methods are at the core of strengths-based CBT (Padesky & Mooney, 2012), which we pioneered at our center and have taught to thousands of therapists around the world. The authors have creatively adapted these concepts and developed exercises well suited to therapist development.

Experiencing CBT from the Inside Out is an ideal guide to help you achieve a more sophisticated understanding of CBT practice. It offers a map for self-discovery and learning. It is up to you to explore the various roads described; the choices you make will help determine what you learn. I suggest you stroll, rather than sprint, through the book. The more time you spend on each chapter, the more opportunities you will have to discover the unexpected. Along the way, your efforts are likely to kindle new depths of meaning and new ways of being to help you become a better therapist and a happier person.

The authors invite you to participate in SP/SR with an open curiosity. I am confident that when you do, you will unearth a genuine appreciation and excitement about all the possibilities CBT offers.

CHRISTINE A. PADESKY, PhD
Center for Cognitive Therapy,
Huntington Beach, California
www.padesky.com

References

Bennett-Levy, J., & Padesky, C. A. (2014). Use it or lose it: Post-workshop reflection enhances learning and utilization of CBT skills. *Cognitive and Behavioral Practice, 21*, 12–19.

Padesky, C. A., & Mooney, K. A. (2012). Strengths-based cognitive-behavioral therapy: A four-step model to build resilience. *Clinical Psychology and Psychotherapy, 19*, 283–290.

Prologue

Welcome to *Experiencing CBT from the Inside Out*. After 15 years of research, self-practice/self-reflection (SP/SR) has reached a level of maturity where we feel confident enough to publish the first publicly available SP/SR workbook. This will enable aspiring and experienced cognitive-behavioral therapists not just to read about CBT but to practice it on themselves. Studies indicate that SP/SR deepens therapists' understanding of CBT and hones their therapeutic skills—including metacompetencies such as reflective skill and capacity to enhance the therapeutic relationship.

In *Experiencing CBT from the Inside Out*, we have taken the opportunity not just to reflect contemporary understandings of CBT, but to extend them. During the course of writing the workbook, we developed the disk model as an integrative way to formulate and contrast *Old* and *New Ways of Being*. While we wrote, we pondered whether an SP/SR workbook was the right place to introduce new ways of doing CBT. But the *Ways of Being* disk model insistently grew, and in the end we were unable to suppress a set of ideas that were bursting to get out.

We invite you, the SP/SR participant, to experiment with this new model while you engage with the workbook; to explore its implications—not just for your understanding of CBT and for the development of your therapeutic skills, but, most of all, for yourself. If in the process you find new ways to extend the model, please let us know. We would be delighted to hear about them.

Most of all, we hope you enjoy experiencing CBT from an inside-out perspective; that the workbook stimulates you; and that it enables you to appreciate the richness and diversity of CBT. One of the great things about CBT is that it has constantly evolved during its relatively brief life. We hope that the *Ways of Being* disk model, and the practice of SP/SR, represent another small step in its evolution.

JAMES BENNETT-LEVY
RICHARD THWAITES
BEVERLY HAARHOFF
HELEN PERRY

For additional information on SP/SR,
visit the program's website:
http://self-practiceself-reflection.com

Acknowledgments

Our great appreciation goes to a number of coauthors and colleagues who in one way or another have supported the growth of SP/SR over the past 15 years. They include Mark Freeston, Nicole Lee, Anna Chaddock, Melanie Davis, Sonja Pohlmann, Elizabeth Hamernik, Katrina Travers, Rick Turner, Michelle Smith, Bethany Paterson, Taryn Beaty, Sarah Farmer, Melanie Fennell, Ann Hackmann, James Hawkins, Bev Taylor, Paul Farrand, Marie Chellingsworth, Craig Chigwedere, Anton-Rupert Laireiter, Ulrike Willutski, Alec Grant, Clare Rees, Kathryn Schneider, Païvi Niemi, Juhani Tiuraniemi, Niccy Fraser, Jan Wilson, Samantha Spafford, Derek Milne, Paul Cromarty, and Peter Armstrong. We also wish to thank Angie Cucchi and the SP/SR participants in Cumbria and Auckland who provided valuable feedback on earlier drafts of the new SP/SR workbook. Our particular thanks and love go to our partners, Judy, Sarah, Errol, and David, who have borne the brunt of the unsocial hours we have devoted to writing. We acknowledge the vast contribution made by Christine A. Padesky to contemporary CBT, and are very appreciative that she so generously agreed to write the Foreword. Finally, many thanks go to a number of staff members at The Guilford Press for their great service and support, in particular Senior Production Editor Jeannie Tang; copyeditor Philip Holthaus; Managing Editor Judith Grauman for her flexibility and care in shepherding the book through its production phase; and Senior Editor Kitty Moore, who has provided wonderful encouragement and support for this project from the first minutes of our meeting in San Francisco.

Contents

CHAPTER 1

Introducing *Experiencing CBT from the Inside Out*

> To fully understand the process of the therapy, there is no substitute
> for using cognitive therapy methods on oneself.
> —CHRISTINE A. PADESKY, p. 288[1]

Research over the past 15 years has consistently shown the positive impact of self-practice/self-reflection (SP/SR) on the skills of CBT practitioners at all levels of experience, from novice to experienced supervisor. We hope that you will enjoy the SP/SR approach; that your cognitive-behavioral therapy (CBT) understanding, skills, confidence, and reflective capacity will benefit from the experience; that SP/SR will be valuable to you at both a professional and personal level; and that your experience will be of direct benefit to your clients. The participant quotes at the beginning of the book are a small sample of the enthusiastic response to SP/SR that has been a consistent feature of the programs that we have facilitated.

In this chapter, we give a brief introduction to SP/SR, discuss the rationale for the SP/SR approach, touch briefly on the research findings, and provide an initial guide to help you navigate the rest of the book. Chapters 2–4 provide additional detail to enhance the experience of SP/SR participants and facilitators.

What Is SP/SR?

SP/SR is an experiential training strategy that provides therapists with a structured experience of using CBT on themselves (SP) and reflecting on that experience (SR). In an SP/SR program, you choose either a professional or a personal problem to focus on, and use CBT strategies to identify, formulate, and address the problem. After the CBT self-practice, you reflect on your experience of the techniques. These reflections appear to be much more valuable if they are written down, rather than simply "thought about," so written reflections are a core part of SP/SR. Reflection happens at various levels; for instance, SP/SR participants may first reflect on their personal experience of a CBT technique (e.g., a behavioral experiment), and identify what elements were helpful (or unhelpful); then they may consider the implications of their experience for their clinical practice, and for their understanding of CBT theory.

If it is a group SP/SR program, participants may share their reflections on the process with colleagues, enabling them to see in what ways their experiences of particular strategies are similar or different from each other. It is this self-experiential element of SP/SR training that differentiates it from other more "usual" forms of CBT training,[2] and typically leads participants to report a "deeper sense of knowing" CBT,[3] having experienced it "from the inside out."

Rationale for SP/SR and Research Findings

In its early stages (mid-1970s to late 1980s), CBT was portrayed as a largely technical intervention with little or no attention paid to "person of the therapist." However, in the 1990s increasing recognition was given to the value of practicing CBT on oneself.[1, 4–7] The reasons given fell into two main categories: first, trainers such as Judith S. Beck and Christine A. Padesky suggested that self-practice of CBT would facilitate CBT skill acquisition and refinement.[1, 5] Second, the publication of two seminal books in 1990, *Cognitive Therapy for Personality Disorders*[4] and *Interpersonal Processes in Cognitive Therapy*,[8] led to a growing realization that therapist self-awareness and self-knowledge is as important in CBT as it is in other therapies[7]— particularly when working with more complex clients where issues often arise in the therapeutic relationship. The words of these writers, together with our own personal experience of using CBT techniques on ourselves,[9] inspired us to develop the original SP/SR workbooks.

Since then, other writers have highlighted the value of self-experience of CBT and self-reflection,[10–12] and a significant body of empirical SP/SR research has emerged.[2, 3, 13–33] The consistent finding across studies in different countries with different groups of participants is that SP/SR enhances understanding of CBT, CBT skills, confidence as a therapist, and belief in the value of CBT as an effective therapy.[16, 17] This research suggests that the impact of SP/SR appears to be as valuable for experienced therapists as it is for novice therapists.[13, 15] Participants report that SP/SR gives them "a deeper sense of knowing" of the therapy through "experiencing CBT from the inside out."[3, 13] The impact is felt in their conceptual skills (e.g., CBT formulation),[18] their technical skills (e.g., ability to utilize CBT techniques more effectively),[13] and interpersonal skills (e.g., empathy for the client).[16, 26, 34, 35] Participants also report that their reflective skills are enhanced through SP/SR.[13] This is an important finding since reflection is a key metacognitive competency that "provides the engine for lifelong learning" throughout a therapist's career.[14, 34]

Perhaps the most significant finding, which emerges as central in every SP/SR study, is that participants consistently report that SP/SR affects their attitude toward clients, enhancing their interpersonal skills and their therapeutic relationships.[22] Through experiencing CBT from the inside out, they gain a firsthand appreciation of the difficulties of change; of the role that underlying patterns such as avoidance, negative cognitive bias, ruminative thinking, and safety behaviors play in maintaining unhelpful ways of being; of the anxiety provoked by some CBT techniques in the service of change (e.g., exposure, behavioral experiments); and of the value of the therapeutic relationship in supporting the change process. CBT training has traditionally been strong at teaching formulation skills and technical skills, but perhaps rather weaker in the interpersonal domain.[36] Experienced CBT therapists report that they have found that the best ways to acquire and refine their interpersonal skills is through self-experience of therapeutic techniques and self-reflection.[37] SP/SR seems to provide a safe and effective vehicle to enhance interpersonal skills in CBT— "a useful middle path between personal therapy and no experiential work, which is acceptable to institutions, practitioners and students" (p. 155).[13]

We suggest that SP/SR has the potential to play a unique role in therapist training and development. We have come to see it as an integrative training strategy that links the declarative understandings of CBT with procedural skills; integrates the interpersonal with the conceptual and the technical; and enhances the channels of communication between the "therapist self" and the "personal self."[16] The self-experiential element of SP/SR facilitates the links; reflection provides the glue.

An Initial Orientation to *Experiencing CBT from the Inside Out*

There is now a whole family of "CBTs" with a number of branches[38] (e.g., cognitive therapy, rational-emotive behavior therapy, schema therapy, acceptance and commitment therapy, low-intensity CBT, metacognitive therapy, and mindfulness-based cognitive therapy). The CBT of *Experiencing CBT from the Inside Out* is focused on the cognitive therapy of Aaron T. Beck, while at times extending this into new methods of formulation. In *Experiencing CBT from the Inside Out,* we have not included techniques from other CBT-influenced therapies such as mindfulness-based cognitive therapy, acceptance and commitment therapy, schema therapy, and metacognitive therapy because some of these will be the subject of separate workbooks in the Guilford Press series *Self-Practice/Self-Reflection Guides for Psychotherapists.*

Experiencing CBT from the Inside Out is organized into two main sections: the introductory chapters (Chapters 1–4), and the SP/SR modules themselves (Modules 1–12). We suggest that all participants read Chapters 1, 2, and 3. Chapter 2 discusses the conceptual underpinnings that have influenced the content of the workbook. Readers will find novel as well as traditional CBT approaches in *Experiencing CBT from the Inside Out*. Our approach to CBT has been influenced by cognitive science, clinical innovations, and neuroscientific understandings that have not yet been fully absorbed into the mainstream. Chapter 2 discusses the rationale for some of the more innovative strategies that you will be experiencing, including the *Ways of Being* model, which provides the core structure of the workbook.

It is important that all SP/SR participants read Chapter 3, "Guidance for SP/SR Participants." This chapter provides guidelines for using the workbook and addresses issues such as how to choose a professional or personal problem to focus on; when to do SP/SR; the pros and cons of doing SP/SR individually or in a group; guidance on how to build your reflective capacity; and how much time to give to SP/SR. This chapter provides instructions for preparing yourself and engaging with the Modules 1–12 that follow. The modules build upon each other in terms of content and theoretical structure. The first six modules (Part I) are focused on "Identifying and Understanding *Unhelpful (Old) Ways of Being*." The second six modules (Part II) use the Part I platform for "Creating and Strengthening *New Ways of Being*." We would like to be able to tell you that there are shortcuts, but the truth is that to get the most out of the workbook, it is best to work through it systematically, giving each module adequate time—an average of about 2 hours in Part I, and more like 3 hours in Part II.

Chapter 4, "Guidance for SP/SR Facilitators" is specifically written for CBT therapists planning to facilitate an SP/SR program. You might be facilitating a peer group; or leading a training group that is doing the program for professional development purposes; or you may be planning to integrate *Experiencing CBT from the Inside Out* with an existing CBT training program. Chapter 4 addresses key issues for running effective SP/SR training programs. It is optional reading for those who are doing *Experiencing CBT from the Inside Out* as SP/SR participants.

Experiencing CBT from the Inside Out is not a conventional CBT textbook. In the modules, we provide materials and examples, but not detailed instructions for the CBT techniques that you will be practicing on yourself. It is assumed that either you will already know the techniques, or will have sufficient knowledge to use the module notes and references to refresh your memory and to guide you. For each module, we have provided Module Notes that you can find at the end of the book, just before the References. Here you will find reference to other books or chapters, which provide more detail about specific strategies featured in the modules. In the workbook we have also "created" three therapists of different levels of experience—Shelly, Jayashri, and David—who have the type of therapist or personal issues that participants typically bring to SP/SR. We provide examples of Shelly's, Jayashri's, and David's SP/SR to help guide your use of specific techniques.

We hope that you enjoy the workbook; that you are able to create for yourself *New Ways of Being* that have a positive impact on your professional and personal life; and that your effectiveness with your clients is considerably enhanced as a result.

CHAPTER 2

Experiencing CBT from the Inside Out: The Conceptual Framework

The purpose of this chapter is to articulate the conceptual framework and influences that have determined the content of *Experiencing CBT from the Inside Out,* and to highlight current developments in CBT that we have incorporated in the content. As an SP/SR participant, it is not essential to read this chapter in order to benefit from the program. However, if you want to understand the rationale for some of the innovative strategies in this workbook, then this chapter should be of interest.

Since 1998, we have created a number of iterations of the original SP/SR workbook, together with colleagues. For the present workbook, we decided to start afresh because the landscape of CBT has changed considerably over recent years. In designing the new workbook, we have endeavored to create a balance between well-recognized and researched Beckian strategies (such as formulation, thought records, behavioral experiments, and Socratic questioning) and a contemporary orientation that acknowledges:

- The importance of process, as well as content of thought.
- The growing influence of transdiagnostic approaches.
- The value of strengths-based strategies.
- The role of culture in shaping our experience of ourselves and the world.
- The central role of experiential strategies in creating change.
- The growing recognition that the body and emotion are intimately related.
- The discovery that body-focused interventions can have a direct impact on emotion, thought, and behavior.

Some of these ideas are encapsulated in two key models from cognitive science that provide the theoretical framework for *Experiencing CBT from the Inside Out*: John D. Teasdale and Philip J. Barnard's Interacting Cognitive Subsystems model[39–44] and Chris Brewin's Retrieval Competition model.[45] We discuss these models in the second half of the chapter. We also acknowledge the influence of Christine A. Padesky and Kathleen A. Mooney, and Kees Korrelboom and colleagues, who have developed innovative CBT interventions that are highly compatible with Teasdale and Barnard's and Brewin's theories. These four sets of authors have led us to introduce into *Experiencing CBT from the Inside Out* a new concept that we describe as the *Ways of Being* (WoB) model. The WoB model may be unfamiliar to CBT therapists, though elements will be recognized from other approaches, particularly those of Padesky and Mooney,[46–48] Korrelboom,[49–53] and Hackmann, Bennett-Levy, and Holmes.[54]

This chapter is divided into three sections. In the first section, we identify some traditional and contemporary concepts in CBT that have framed the development of *Experiencing CBT from the Inside Out*, and give a rationale for their inclusion. In the second section, we discuss the conceptual and clinical influences on the development of the *WoB* model. In the final section, we describe the rationale for the *WoB* model and its key features.

Key CBT Concepts in *Experiencing CBT from the Inside Out*

The Central Role of Formulation in CBT

Underpinning all elements of *Experiencing CBT from the Inside Out*, including the *WoB* model, is a principle that has been central to CBT since its inception: the pivotal role of formulation.[10, 11, 55–57] Beckian CBT has always had a reputation for being theoretically coherent, but "methodologically permissive."[58] This approach has allowed creativity to flourish and spawned a whole family of CBT offshoots (e.g., schema therapy, acceptance and commitment therapy, metacognitive therapy, and mindfulness-based cognitive therapy). We have aimed to be true to this heritage by making formulation the "spine" of the workbook, while being "methodologically permissive" with old and new ideas.

A Focus on Process and Underlying Patterns of Thought and Behavior, as Well as Content of Thoughts

Early versions of CBT tended to have a primary focus on changing the content of thoughts and modifying "dysfunctional ways" of thinking and behaving. However, even though in early versions of CBT *process* played second fiddle to *content*, CBT has always recognized the importance of underlying patterns of behavior (e.g., avoidance) and unhelpful thinking styles (e.g., catastrophization) in maintaining problems.[57, 59]

Since the turn of the century, there has been a progressively greater emphasis on the *processes* that drive thoughts and maintain behavior, which has led to the development of new forms of therapy (e.g., mindfulness-based cognitive therapy, metacognitive therapy, acceptance and commitment therapy) that focus more on the client's *relationship* to thoughts, (and emotions, body, and behavior), rather than the actual *content* of thought. This focus on underlying patterns of thought and behavior was highlighted in a landmark book by Alison G. Harvey, Edward Watkins, Warren Mansell, and Roz Shafran (2004), *Cognitive Behavioural Processes across Psychological Disorders.*[60] These authors recognized that processes such as self-focused attention, avoidance of painful memories, faulty reasoning processes such as all-or-nothing thinking, thought suppression, rumination, safety-seeking behaviors, behavioral avoidance, and other underlying patterns tended to be common across disorders.

Experiencing CBT from the Inside Out has therefore emphasized *process* as well as *content* of thought (see, e.g., Modules 4 and 5), and sought to direct participants' attention to their underlying patterns of thought and behavior.

A Transdiagnostic Approach

In its development, CBT has been closely tied to psychiatric diagnosis: Beck and colleagues developed specific treatment manuals for depression and anxiety,[57, 59] and over the following years, specific treatments were developed for a range of psychiatric disorders, reflected in books such as Keith Hawton, David Clark, Paul Salkovskis, and Joan Kirk's (1989) *Cognitive Behaviour Therapy for Psychiatric Problems*[61] and Salkovksis's (1996) *Frontiers of Cognitive Therapy.*[62] However, in recent years, we have started to see a move toward a transdiagnostic emphasis in CBT foreshadowed by Harvey et al.'s book,[60] which was subtitled *A Transdiagnostic Approach to Research and Treatment.* In recent times CBT therapists,[63–65] spearheaded by David H. Barlow and colleagues, have started to develop transdiagnostic treatment protocols with promising results.[66, 67]

SP/SR workbooks have always been designed for training rather than therapy, and so from the outset have had a transdiagnostic emphasis, with a focus on the self-practice of CBT techniques. *Experiencing CBT from the Inside Out* retains the transdiagnostic emphasis of previous workbooks. However, we observe that there is now greater alignment between this transdiagnostic emphasis of SP/SR and recent directions in CBT.

A Strengths-Based Approach

The traditional focus of CBT has been to elicit and formulate the problem, particularly by identifying unhelpful thoughts and behaviors, and then work to modify thinking and develop more adaptive behaviors in order to address the problem successfully. The effectiveness of this strategy has been repeatedly demonstrated.

However, in recent years, there has also been an increasing focus on incorporating client strengths into CBT, exemplified in the work of Christine Padesky and colleagues.[11, 46, 48] As Kuyken, Padesky, and Dudley have written, "Conceptualization that attends to client strengths . . . has a number of advantages. It provides a description and understanding of the whole person, not just problematic issues. A strengths focus broadens potential therapy outcomes from alleviation of distress and resumption of normal functioning to improvement of the client's quality of life and bolstering client resilience" (p. 8).[11] The parallel growth of evidence-based interventions from positive psychology,[68–72] and recent empirical data indicate that a strengths-based CBT approach may actually have advantages over a deficit-focused model.[73,74] This suggests that the movement toward a greater emphasis on strengths in CBT may well be justified.

Accordingly, in *Experiencing CBT from the Inside Out*, strengths are explicitly incorporated into the CBT formulation and are used to facilitate and support the *New Ways of Being*.

A Culturally Responsive Therapy

CBT was developed in a Western cultural setting, and until recently little attention was given to the relevance of CBT cross-culturally, or to the influence of culture on the effectiveness of CBT. Furthermore, although cultural mores and traditions clearly have a significant influence on people's thinking and ways of being in the world, CBT formulations have not usually included cultural influences. Recently, clinicians have sought to develop culturally responsive adaptations of CBT,[75–78] and are starting to generate CBT research with different cultural groups,[79–81] including the use of transdiagnostic approaches.[82]

Patricia Hays has been at the forefront in introducing a cultural perspective into CBT,[75, 83, 84] and has provided a broad definition of culture, summarized in the acronym ADDRESSING.[75] These cultural influences are:

Age and generational influences.
Developmental and other physical, cognitive, sensory, and psychiatric **D**isabilities.
Religion and spiritual orientation.
Ethnic and racial identity.
Socioeconomic status.
Sexual orientation.
Indigenous heritage.
National origin.
Gender.

Recognizing the importance of culture in shaping our experience of the world, *Experiencing CBT from the Inside Out* has included a place for cultural influences in the CBT formulations in Module 2.

The Cognitive Science Foundations of the Ways of Being (WoB) Model

Two models from cognitive science have been highly influential in developing our approach to CBT, reflected in the *WoB* model: Teasdale and Barnard's Interacting Cognitive Subsystems (ICS)[39–44, 99, 100] and Brewin's Retrieval Competition account of CBT.[45] Their theoretically derived proposals for creating effective therapeutic change are compelling, and their models are largely complementary.

ICS is a complex model, which we simplify here by highlighting only those aspects that are relevant to the present purposes. The reader should consult Teasdale, Barnard, and other authors who have written about ICS to gain a fuller understanding. In brief, Teasdale and Barnard posit two information-processing "systems": a propositional system and an implicational system. The features of these two systems that are relevant to the *WoB* model are set out in the table on page 10.

ICS suggests that the two systems have quite different qualities. Propositional knowledge is explicit and conveys specific information (e.g., "I need more knowledge and skills to treat clients with bipolar disorder"). Propositional knowledge has no direct linkage with bodily experience, emotion, or sensory input. Its truth value can be tested and verified (intellectual knowing). In contrast, the implicational system is schematic and holistic. It is often experienced as a "felt sense"; input from the body, from emotions, and from sensory information form a central part of the "schema package," creating implicit meanings that are not always verbalizable (e.g., therapists may on occasions experience a felt sense of hopelessness when working with severely depressed clients). These felt senses are not directly testable, and are experienced as heart-level emotional beliefs (e.g., "I know intellectually that I do some good with depressed clients, but I never feel like I do").

Teasdale and Barnard's model has direct implications for treatment. It suggests that for significant change to occur, rational disputational interventions and psychoeducation tend to be inadequate, unless they lead to a significant perspective shift (an "alternative schematic model" in Teasdale and Barnard's terms); see the table on page 10. For instance, it has been found that, while both thought records and behavioral experiments shed light on awareness and understanding of the problem, behavioral experiments tend to be rather more effective than thought records in producing change.[85, 86] The ICS model suggests that experiential interventions such as behavioral experiments, imagery-based interventions, adopting new bodily postures embodying strength or competence, cultivating a "mindful" relationship to thoughts and emotions, or developing a "compassionate mind" will tend to have a direct impact on the implicational system, due to their impact at all levels of a schema (body, emotion, cognition, behavior). The ICS model also suggests that adopting a different mind-set (e.g., a *New Ways of Being* mind-set) as a frame of reference for processing the impact of experiential strategies is likely to facilitate change, whereas processing experiences through the lens of the *Old Ways of Being* will not. For instance, if a male client, who is phobic of public speaking, processes a successful talk through his *Old Ways of Being* lens, he is likely to draw the conclusion

SUMMARY OF KEY ELEMENTS OF TEASDALE AND BARNARD'S ICS MODEL

Propositional System	Implicational System
Phenomenology within the ICS Model	
Propositional meaning is able to be represented linguistically and conveys specific information in the form of explicit knowledge (e.g., "I did a poor assessment with that client").	Implicational meanings are schematic, holistic, and cross-situational. They are experienced as implicit "felt senses" and are often difficult to put into words (e.g., "my sense of uselessness as a therapist" or, at a less generalized level, "my heartsink when really depressed clients enter the room").
There is no direct input to the propositional system from the body, from emotions, or from sensory experience.	Body, emotions, and sensory input (e.g., smell, tone of voice) carry implicit meanings. All are intrinsic to the "schema package." Any of them may trigger activation of the schema (e.g., fatigue or a critical-sounding voice).
Propositional knowledge has truth value, which can be rationally evaluated and verified by evidence (e.g., "What did I do well? What did I do poorly?"). It is experienced as "head-level" intellectual belief.	Implicational schema have a holistic "felt sense" of rightness. They cannot be evaluated as true or false (e.g., "It's just how I am"). They are experienced as "heart-level" or "gut-level" emotional beliefs.
Implications for Treatment within the ICS Model	
Rational disputation interventions (e.g., thought records) and psychoeducation are more likely to impact only on the propositional system, and are therefore less likely than experiential strategies to create cross-situational *New Ways of Being*. However, there are exceptions in cases where (1) new information leads to new higher-level meanings (e.g., an unconfident novice therapist discovering from his supervisor that many clients do not improve through short-term therapy leading him to reevaluate his level of competence); (2) where rationally based interventions lead to the creation of new "schematic models" (e.g., "I've discovered that my thoughts are not facts; they are ideas and opinions which can be considered and examined").	Experiential interventions (e.g., behavioral experiments, imagery, modifying bodily postures, mindfulness meditation, attentional retraining and compassion-focused approaches) are more likely than rationally based interventions to impact at the implicational level, and therefore to create *New Ways of Being*. This is due to their direct impact at the schematic level (emotion, body, cognition, behavior). The potential for change is particularly enhanced if challenging situations are approached with a new, more adaptive mind-set (in Teasdale's terms, a new or modified "schematic model")—for example, "I'm a therapist-in-training. I am learning as I go."

that he "got away with it," which would be unlikely to assist the process of change. On the other hand, if he processes it through his *New Ways of Being* perspective—"I am a competent public speaker (even though I might not believe it much at the moment)"—he would regard the talk as building evidence for this new idea about himself.

Brewin's[45] retrieval competition account of CBT seeks to clarify the relationship between old and new "memory representations," or in Teasdale and Barnard's terms, the relationship between "alternative schematic models." Brewin proposes that when clients have emotional disorders, negative memory representations (schema) are highly accessible with intrusive memories, self-depreciating interpretations, and ruminative thoughts dominating (e.g., "I'm useless" memories). It is assumed that both positive and negative memory representations are in "retrieval competition" (the negative memory representations are never "extinguished," merely rendered less accessible).

The aim of CBT is therefore to facilitate the retrieval of alternative adaptive memories (e.g., "times when I've shown my worth") by enhancing and strengthening the accessibility of those memories, so that they are activated across a wide range of situations and win the retrieval competition. As with the ICS model, the adoption of a *New Ways of Being* perspective is likely to enhance accessibility of positive memory representations, and make them more available in future situations.

In the *WoB* model described below, we have aimed to capture key elements of the ICS and retrieved competition models. Specifically we note the value of:

1. Developing an "alternative schematic model" or mind-set (i.e., the *New Ways of Being*).
2. Interpreting new experiences from a *New Ways of Being* perspective.
3. Formulating and contrasting the unhelpful *Old Ways of Being* and the *New Ways of Being* that are in retrieval competition.
4. Using behavioral experiments, imagery, and other experiential techniques to strengthen *New Ways of Being*.
5. Embodying the *New Ways of Being*, using body-oriented interventions (e.g., adopting a bodily posture of strength and confidence).

Clinical Influences on the Ways of Being Model

The clinical innovations of two groups of CBT clinicians, Christine Padesky and Kathleen Mooney and Kees Korreboom and colleagues, have had a significant influence on the *WoB* model. Padesky and Mooney's Old System/New System approach was primarily developed in relation to clients with chronic difficulties who were not responding to classic CBT interventions, especially clients with personality disorders, who have inflexible negative core beliefs.[47, 87] The aim of their approach is to transform "old systems" of interacting in the world into more adaptive "new systems." Therapists and clients co-construct a vision of how the person would like to be and how he or she would like others to be. This vision is developed in words, imagery, kinesthetic body awareness, metaphors, and related memories. Then new core beliefs, underlying assumptions, and behavioral strategies that support those new ways of being are identified. Korrelboom, working in an inpatient clinical setting, has developed COMET— COmpetitive MEmory Training—for patients with low self-esteem who may have diagnoses such as personality disorder, depression, and eating disorders.[49–53, 88] The goal of COMET is to establish and strengthen a positive self-image in these patients.

Both Padesky and Mooney's Old System/New System approach and Korrelboom's COMET self-image training start by formulating the current negative state (Old System/

negative self-image), before constructing a positive alternative (New System/credible positive self-image). Both strategies use imagery to establish the positive alternative. Thereafter they emphasize slightly different techniques to strengthen confidence in the New System/positive self-image. Padesky and Mooney give particular weight to role plays and behavioral experiments[87]; Korrelboom tends to favor positive imagery rehearsal and sensory (music) and body-oriented ways to strengthen the new perspective.

The fit between Teasdale and Barnard's and Brewin's theories, and Padesky and Mooney's and Korrelboom's innovative strategies are clear: all suggest the importance of creating "alternative schematic models"[40, 44] and processing new experiences through these lenses, with the goal of increasing their salience and accessibility for future use. Additionally Teasdale and Barnard, Padesky and Mooney, and Korrelboom all place great weight on "arranging for experiences in which new or modified models are created" (p. 90),[39] such as behavioral experiments, imagery rehearsal, or other enactive procedures such as Korrelboom's sensory- and body-oriented strategies. Recent empirical literature points to an increased awareness of the potential impact on cognition, emotion, and relationships of body-oriented interventions.[101–104]

Description and Key Features of the Ways of Being Model

Rationale for the Ways of Being Model and Description

The first time that one of us used the term *"New Ways of Being"* in a publication was in Hackmann et al.'s *Oxford Guide to Imagery in Cognitive Therapy*.[54] Hackmann et al. used *"New Ways of Being"* to refer to "a positive orientation that clients, who had previously had strong, persistent negative beliefs, are encouraged to develop towards themselves. . . . New ways of Being encompass a variety of new cognitions, behaviors, emotions, physiological reactions, and felt senses" (p. 182). The *Ways of Being* model thus identifies that the change from old to new ways of being happens at a multimodal schematic level, consistent with Teasdale and Barnard's ICS approach. Hackmann et al. added: "It is usually essential to validate current dysfunctional ways of being as understandable and adaptive responses to past circumstances, before moving on to the construction of alternatives. However, the principal focus of new ways of being therapy work is on envisioning new ways of being or desired states" (p. 182).

In *Experiencing CBT from the Inside Out*, we have used the idea of *Old (Unhelpful) Ways of Being* and *New Ways of Being* to give coherence to the workbook and provide an overall framework: the first six modules (Part I of the workbook) are focused on identifying and understanding the *Old/Unhelpful Ways of Being*; Part II is focused on creating *New Ways of Being*. However, since the introduction of the *New Ways of Being* concept in the Hackmann et al. book, we have come to realize that schema change does not necessarily involve core belief change, as implied by much of the CBT literature. Ian James, Matt Goodman, and Katharina Reichelt[90] have recently remarked that such a view is "rather monodimensional." Our clinical experience supports this conclusion. James et al. use examples from sports psychology to illustrate how a professional golfer wanting to change his or her technique will need to spend many hours practicing the new swing. The task is to weaken the old schemas and establish new ones. Repetition involves creating new neural networks that can be modified over time. Multimodal schema change is central to the process, but there is no implication of core belief change. How is change achieved? James et al. write: "This might involve the use of imagery, behavioural retraining, body posture retraining, memory reconditioning techniques" (p. 8).[90] These are all strategies that we have incorporated into the *New Ways of Being* model that is featured in Modules 9–11.

Our recent experience of using the *WoB* model with SP/SR participants, and with some of our clients, is that it is as relevant for people without strong negative core beliefs or major personality issues, as it is for more distressed clients. Indeed, we have purposely chosen not to introduce core beliefs into the workbook exercises, partly because we do not want or expect SP/SR participants to go this "deep," and partly because, as Ian James[91] pointed out some time ago, the evidence base is that clients do well in short-term CBT therapy without doing core belief work, and at times it may actually be countertherapeutic for therapists to do schema work with clients in short-term therapy.

To illustrate this point further: many of us have "stuck" beliefs about ourselves (e.g., "I'm no good at working with people who are aggressive"; "I'm so disorganized!") that are firmly held, but do not indicate major psychopathology or dysfunctional core beliefs. Therapeutically significant perspective shifts may occur without the need to address issues at a core belief level. For instance, it is now well documented that clients may experience a perspective shift by developing a different relationship to their thoughts through distancing or mindfulness strategies.[92] Thoughts are no longer "facts," but opinions, ideas, or transient cognitive experiences open to validation or invalidation. As an example in the therapist context, novice therapists are often under the illusion that they are incompetent because some clients are not improving. Informing them that significant numbers of clients fail to attend appointments and/or do not "recover" regardless of the expertise of the therapist can lead to a perspective shift that normalizes their expectations, and significantly reduces anxiety levels and feelings of incompetence. In other words, the perspective shift may initiate a *New Way of Being:* "I'm doing all right as I am, and my competency is continuing to develop," which can be strengthened over time.

In summary, the *WoB* model is a transdiagnostic, strengths-based approach, which emphasizes the value of experiential techniques in promoting change. The idea of *Old* and *New Ways of Being* is readily applicable to people without major psychopathology, who have "stuck" beliefs or patterns of thought or behavior. They may benefit from CBT strategies that create a perspective shift, leading to a change in the relative salience and accessibility of alternative *Ways of Being*. For a workbook directed toward therapists looking to make changes in their professional or personal lives over 12 modules, *Ways of Being* seems a useful model.

The Disk Model Representation of *Old (Unhelpful)* and *New Ways of Being*

Alongside the *WoB* model, we have introduced a new way of representing the relationship between thoughts, behavior, and emotions/bodily sensations: a disk model of three concentric circles (see Module 9, pages 192–193 and 195–196). Teasdale and Barnard's ICS suggests that at the implicational level of "felt sense," the boundaries between bodily experience, emotions, cognitions, and behaviors are closely merged. Teasdale further suggests that old minds are "wheeled out" as a package, and new minds are "wheeled in" as circumstances change (p. 101).[39] The disk model seems to us to represent the holistic nature of the ICS/*Ways of Being* rather better than traditional formulation diagrams (e.g., in Module 2); there is a sense that it can be more easily "wheeled in" and "wheeled out" as a gestalt; and it has the added advantage of being easier to visualize and memorize.

One other feature of the disk model that should be noted is that personal strengths have been included at the base of the *New Ways of Being* model. This inclusion in the *New Ways* model (but not the *Old*) is for the obvious reason that personal strengths play a central role in the creation and development of *New Ways of Being*.

Concluding Comments

One of the most exciting features of CBT over the past 40 years has been its constant evolution, driven by theory and supported by empirical research, and encouraged by the eagerness of the CBT community to celebrate innovation. In constructing a new SP/SR workbook for CBT therapists, we have wanted not just to reflect what has gone before, but to incorporate contemporary perspectives that might stand the test of time—at least for the next few years! We recognize that some readers might think we have gone too far by not only reflecting on but suggesting new perspectives; others may consider that we have not gone far enough, for instance, by not including mindfulness exercises. Certainly, we hope the ideas in *Experiencing CBT from the Inside Out* contribute to healthy debate. If they do, it will have served one of its purposes.

As we stated at the start of this chapter, formulation is the bedrock of Beckian CBT, and we hope that *Experiencing CBT from the Inside Out* reflects our appreciation of its continued importance. Similarly, our respect for theory and for clinical innovation has driven the content of *Experiencing CBT from the Inside Out*. Above all, our interest in developing this workbook is to give participants an appreciation of CBT techniques from the inside—in particular experiential techniques, which we regard as the primary catalysts of change—and to facilitate a journey that is both professionally and personally valuable. It is by these criteria that the success or otherwise of this workbook will be judged.

CHAPTER 3

Guidance for SP/SR Participants

This chapter is essential reading for anyone engaging with SP/SR as a participant. It poses key questions for you to consider prior to starting the program, and provides guidelines for getting the greatest benefit from the experience. It is also an important chapter for SP/SR facilitators, trainers, and supervisors as it informs much of the content of Chapter 4.

Over the past decade SP/SR participants in different countries have repeatedly expressed how much they have gained from SP/SR. You may have seen a sample of their comments at the front of the book to illustrate the kinds of experience that they report. However, it has also become clear that some participants benefit more than others, and we are now beginning to understand why this is the case. What we have learned is that participants' level of engagement is central to the benefit that they experience from SP/SR.[2, 15, 16, 25] Consequently, the central theme of this chapter is: How can you best prepare for SP/SR in order to maximize engagement and reap the most benefit?

As we indicated in Chapter 1, the kinds of benefits of SP/SR that have been identified encompass increased CBT understanding, skills, and confidence; insights and changes in the "personal self" and the "therapist self"; enhanced reflective capacity; and a more nuanced and individualized approach to individual clients. We cite references in Chapter 1 for you to study the research in more detail if you wish, but it is probably better to approach the workbook without too many preconceptions. We hope that the comments of other participants at the front of the book will give you some confidence that your time and energy will reap rewards.

This chapter is divided into four sections. The first section illustrates how SP/SR can be undertaken in various contexts: on your own, with a buddy, in groups, or with a supervisor. It provides guidance for deriving the most benefit from these different contexts. The next section focuses on practical measures to maximize your engagement with SP/SR: how to choose your "challenging problem"; time management; choosing when to do SP/SR; and keeping yourself safe. A third section is focused specifically on growing your reflective capacity. It is not a "given" that we know how to reflect. This section contains tips for building your reflective skills. These three sections are designed to enhance your engagement with SP/SR and to enable you to get the most benefit from *Experiencing CBT from the Inside Out*. The chapter finishes by introducing you to the three therapists, Shelly, Jayashri, and David, whose examples we use throughout Modules 1–12.

SP/SR Contexts: Self-Guided SP/SR, with a Buddy, in Groups, or with a Supervisor

Tackling the SP/SR Workbook on Your Own

There are many reasons for choosing to work through the SP/SR exercises on your own, for example: geographical or professional isolation; not being willing to or not having the means or ability to use connecting technologies such as the Internet; a personal preference for privacy; or a sense that you work through things better on your own. If this is your preferred option, remember that it is usually more difficult to stick to something when the only person you are accountable to is yourself! Setting aside regular times to engage with the exercises and developing clear goals about what you intend to achieve is very important. You may also find that working through the self-practice exercises can sometimes trigger an unexpected emotional response that is more intense than you may have anticipated; therefore it is worth paying particular attention to developing a Personal Safeguard Strategy in advance if you are working alone. This will be discussed in more detail later in the chapter.

Working through the SP/SR Workbook with a Colleague or "Buddy"

Participant feedback over a number of years has repeatedly confirmed that therapists find that engaging in an SP/SR program is enhanced when the experience is shared.[2, 19] Working through the exercises and then sharing reflections with another person can be a very rewarding experience and can be useful in overcoming some of the difficulties of the more individualized approach. An experience shared helps us to stay on track, facilitates expansion and elaboration of the experience of both SP and SR, normalizes difficulties, and ideally provides support, encouragement, and empathic attunement. However, your choice of partner needs to be a considered one. The level of trust should be high, and confidentiality is obviously of the greatest importance. It is also important to consider relative levels of experience, theoretical knowledge of the CBT model, and stage of professional development. As will be discussed in more detail later, less experienced therapists or therapists who are undertaking basic training are generally advised to focus their attention on developing an understanding of, and skill in applying the CBT model, whereas experienced therapists may be more interested in developing self-understanding at a more personal level in order to work more effectively with complex clients where issues in the therapeutic relationship can assume greater centrality.[12, 35, 93, 94] In a paired situation, therefore, it is important to take these factors into consideration in order to maximize the experience and minimize any possible frustration or disappointment. Finally, make sure that when working with one other person that time is shared equally. Be wary of getting into a situation where one person dominates and the other becomes a passive listener, or a "therapist" to the other.

Using the SP/SR Workbook in Groups

Working through the SP/SR program in a group is an exciting alternative, and feedback confirms that participants experiencing SP/SR in this context enjoy considerable benefits, amplifying many of the advantages of a peer or buddy situation. Groups can be of many types: for example, practitioners working in a mental health center or private practice, peer supervision groups, interest groups, or groups undertaking a university degree program. Groups can meet "physically" or be "virtual" in the sense that interaction is via the Internet where discussion forums, chat rooms, or interactive blogging sites can be established. Some of the previously mentioned factors such as trust, compatibility, level of experience, and so on need to be carefully considered. Pros and cons concerning groups who are in close professional contact with each other also require some consideration and management, as the professional context can inhibit frank disclosure, particularly if the organization is a hierarchical one.

Using the SP/SR Workbook with a Supervisor

The SP/SR workbook can be a very useful addition to "supervision as usual" and may be used in a variety of different ways in this context. Progress through the workbook can become a regular item on the supervision agenda and issues that may arise in relation to the SP/SR workbook can be discussed as needed. This can be a useful and supportive model to consider for therapists interested in working through the modules alone using a self-guided approach.

The workbook can also be used in supervision in a more targeted manner: for example, particular SP exercises could be recommended to enhance understanding and skillful use of those interventions contained in the workbook (many of which are standard CBT interventions such as the activity and mood diary, thought records, and behavioral experiments). In working with more experienced therapists, workbook exercises can be used to facilitate self-understanding relevant to understanding therapeutic relationship ruptures and other difficulties.

Practicalities of SP/SR: Maximizing Engagement and Reaping the Benefits

Choosing the "Challenging Problem"

Working through the SP/SR workbook puts you at center stage. In the first instance, you need to select a "challenging problem" as a starting point for the application of the self-practice exercises. You will receive plenty of guidance in doing this when you start the exercises. You need to consider whether you want to work on a *personal* or a *professional* area of difficulty. As a general guideline, we would suggest that if you are a relatively new therapist, you should consider areas of difficulty relating to your work: quite possibly to your development as a therapist. Areas could be your understanding and application of aspects of the CBT model, your confidence as a therapist, or the competing demands of whatever program you are completing. Situations such as supervision or clinical practice requirements; relationships with your supervisors, mentors, or peers; anxieties around working with certain clients; or doubts about yourself as a therapist are typical examples.

More experienced practitioners, on the other hand, may find that working on personal areas of difficulty is more relevant to working with complex clients, supervision of trainees, or the like. Examples of more personally relevant problems could be interpersonal problems, recognizing an overconcern with what others may think of you, difficulties with certain types of emotional expression such as anger, or finding it difficult to trust other people. There is of course no reason why you should not use the exercises in the workbook to work on more than one issue. This could be done in tandem or in sequence. It is important, however, to monitor yourself, choose what is appropriate to your current needs and available time, and avoid issues which might elicit strong emotional reactions (e.g., current or past traumas, or complicated grief).

Time Management

You will gain most if you work through the 12 modules systematically. Each module builds on what has been achieved in the previous one—you are likely to lose the thread through shortcuts. It is important to set aside sufficient time to work through the exercises, and to reflect on the process.

Establish a routine that works for you. Most people do not have an empty period within their day. If you can, find a way to build a set time for SP/SR into your days. Although much of the work will be carried out in your day-to-day life, it will help to identify a specific time to reflect on and complete the workbook. Maybe it is getting up a little earlier, or, if you have children, after they have gone to bed? You could use a diary or calendar to plan. Leaving long gaps of time between modules or exercises may mean losing focus and interest.

How much time should you set aside? Our experience suggests that each module is best completed over a week if time and space allows. Modules in the first half of the workbook will probably take about 1–2 hours (Module 2 may take 2–3 hours). Modules in the second part (Modules 7–12) may take a bit longer, perhaps 2–3 hours per module. Exercises in some of the modules (e.g., Modules 3, 9, 10, 11) may require daily practice. Taking this into account, your total commitment to the program should cover at least 12 weeks.

If the program is group-based, a module every 2 weeks may be more realistic. This will give the group time both for their self-practice and for personal reflections, and to read and comment upon the reflections of other group members. Recognizing the realistic amount of time needed will reduce the likelihood of being unexpectedly overwhelmed.

Choosing When to Do SP/SR

It is advisable to avoid doing SP/SR at times of high personal stress because it is not designed to be "self-therapy" and can be counterproductive during such times. The danger is that it becomes just another "thing to do," or worse still, it may trigger further distress if you find yourself working on emotionally intense thoughts. Far better to delay your participation to another time, if this is at all possible. If needing to do SP/SR as a course requirement, choose a problem at the mild end of the spectrum.

Keeping Yourself Safe

Ensuring Confidentiality

If you are using the workbook in training, or in a group that meets face-to-face or in a wider Internet-based forum, remember that you are in *total* control of what you share. There are two issues here: reflection in your private space, and reflection in the public space. We encourage you to reflect in depth in your private space (see the section "Building Your Reflective Capacity" in this chapter). In the public space, you should make a clear distinction between the *content* and *process* of your CBT self-practice. Our general recommendation is that in the public space you should reflect on the CBT *process* (e.g., "I found it hard to create a behavioral experiment, but once I did so . . ."), but not on the *content* of your CBT self-practice (e.g., "My anxiety at asking my boss for time off was out of control"). Sometimes when groups have developed close bonds, participants make their own informal decisions about including reflections on content, but these groups tend to be the exceptions.

Developing a Personal Safeguard Strategy

SP/SR is not always comfortable. We can all run across thoughts and feelings that take us by surprise and upset us. This is to be expected and generally resolves fairly quickly through the SP/SR process. However, at times the distress may seem prolonged and less manageable. For this reason we recommend that you develop a *Personal Safeguard Strategy* before you commence the program. By this we mean a series of graded steps you might take if you become distressed during the program. Here is a typical example of a three-step Personal Safeguard Strategy:

1. Discuss the issue with my partner (or an SP/SR colleague).
2. Talk with the SP/SR facilitator (or my supervisor).
3. If my unpleasant or distressing emotional reaction does not resolve over 2 or 3 weeks, see an identified local therapist or my GP.

Maximizing Engagement and Reaping the Benefits of SP/SR

- Choose an appropriate "challenging problem."
- Consider whether this should be a professional or a personal problem.
- Do not choose an area of difficulty relating to current or past trauma.
- Time management: Set aside sufficient time and plan when to do SP/SR.
- Choose when to do SP/SR: Avoid SP/SR at times of high personal stress.
- Keep yourself safe: Establish clear confidentiality agreements.
- Distinguish between your reflections in your private space and reflections in the public space.
- To maintain the sense of safety, the general recommendation is that in the public space you should reflect on the process, but not the content of your self-practice experience.
- Establish a Personal Safeguard Strategy prior to starting SP/SR in case you become distressed during the process.

Building Your Reflective Capacity

Our experience in delivering SP/SR programs suggests that the level of reflective skill and motivation to reflect is variable within the therapist population. Some CBT therapists have what seems like a "natural" reflective capacity from the very start of their training; other therapists may be quite suspicious and/or nervous about reflection, and take longer to engage with an SP/SR program. In addition, home pressures and busy professional lives can make it harder to reflect effectively on a consistent basis. The CBT literature currently provides very little guidance for therapists about how to reflect, so in this section we provide some general guidelines and tips. The guidelines cover preparation for reflection, the process of reflection, self-reflective writing, and how to take care of yourself during the process.

Preparing for Reflection

It is important to establish a structure that facilitates reflection, feels safe, and is manageable and sustainable.

- **Do not wait for a moment when you feel like opening the workbook.** For most people there will always be a list of things that need doing in other areas of your life, so scheduling regular time for reflection is important. See also the section "Time Management" above.

- **Be prepared for strong emotional reactions.** SP/SR can be uncomfortable, distressing, exhilarating, exciting, or joyful. There is no right or wrong way to respond. People have different reactions and you can expect to react differently to different modules.

- **Be prepared for times of ambivalence or thoughts of wanting to give up.** These are normal. Change is difficult. Try not to make rapid decisions about abandoning the program. Use the techniques within the workbook (e.g., problem solving) to troubleshoot and identify whether terminating your involvement in an SP/SR program is the correct decision at that point.

- **Be aware of potential natural breaks in the process** (e.g., vacations) and take action to minimize disruption. Feedback suggests that these are potential risk points for disengagement unless you plan how to maintain continuity and reengagement after a break.

- **Plan where you will keep the workbook and your written reflections.** You might feel somewhat anxious about people reading your workbook reflections. This is similar to the feelings that clients have around keeping thought diaries. Choose where you will keep your workbook or reflections. Some people find that they prefer to keep them electronically so that they are password-protected. Find a solution that works for you and use this as a starting point for thinking about the implications for clients of keeping their personal thoughts in a secure place.

The Process of Reflection

- **Find a time and place** where you are unlikely to be disturbed or distracted.

- **Transition from the self-practice exercise to the task of reflecting.** SP/SR participants typically report that using a focused breathing exercise or a mindfulness exercise is helpful in enabling them to move from the self-practice into a more reflective state.

- **Use whatever works for you to enhance your recall of situations and awareness of your own thoughts and feelings:**
  - You may find it easier to close your eyes when trying to recall a situation and the accompanying emotions, bodily reactions, thoughts, and behaviors.
  - Choose a specific situation and the moments when the situation felt most intense.
  - When you are recalling a situation, reconstruct it in your mind's eye in as much sensory detail as possible (e.g., What was the client wearing, What did the room look like, the atmosphere, the sounds, the smells?).
  - Tune into your body, notice how you are (and were) feeling both physically and emotionally.

- **Stay with your thoughts and feelings**. Often CBT therapists find themselves rushing to challenge their thoughts or to problem-solve. This can be done at the expense of accessing deeper levels of thought or more fully experiencing the emotions that accompany these thoughts. Try not to push thoughts away that feel uncomfortable or perhaps do not fit with how you like to see yourself.

- **Notice the unexpected**. There might be a mismatch between what you notice and what you expected—perhaps this could even be a *lack* of feeling or thinking when you would expect to think or feel something. It may be that you find yourself slipping back into *Old Ways of Being* when you think you have previously changed the old ways of thinking and feeling.

- **Monitor whether you are reflecting or ruminating.** If you catch yourself drifting off or you realize that your thinking is going around in circles, then it is worth considering whether you have slipped from a reflective space (objective, detached) into a more ruminative process.

- **Remain compassionate toward yourself.** Experience tells us that therapists can often express frustration or annoyance when they identify their own unhelpful beliefs or behaviors. On occasions, they may become quite distressed. There can often be an unacknowledged thought along the lines of: "I'm a therapist and spend all day helping people to understand and change themselves; I shouldn't ever think or behave unhelpfully." Therapists are also human beings! We all behave unhelpfully at times; we all have beliefs that are self-limiting or even self-destructive. Noticing your thoughts and behaviors in a curious, accepting, and compassionate way without rushing to judgment is a helpful stance for doing SP/SR.

- **Use SP/SR to address self-critical thoughts**. If you find yourself being self-critical, learning to notice this and bringing your attention back to the focus of the work is likely to be useful. Self-critical thoughts can be valuable SP/SR experiences, leading to insight and change both personally and professionally. We will return to this idea throughout the workbook.

- **Reflection can happen in stages and when you least expect it**. If you find yourself getting stuck, it is fine to put your reflections to one side and revisit them later. It is often the case that something else occurs to you later in the module or workbook, which enables you to come back and expand on your initial reflections.

- **Ask yourself questions as you reflect on your experiences.** The final section of each module has a set of self-reflective questions—but feel free to add your own. The goal is to deepen your understanding and find new links by relating your personal experience to your beliefs about yourself, your clients, and CBT as a model of psychotherapy.

- **Aim to link the personal and the professional.** Our research data suggest that the people who gain most benefit are those who can use SP/SR to reflect both on how they see themselves as therapists and as people in their wider lives.[14, 25] Some of the people who have benefited most have shown a spiraling pattern of back-and-forth reflections between their "therapist self" and "personal self."

Self-Reflective Writing

- **Write in the first person.** When writing your reflections on your practice, it is usually most useful to write in the first person (e.g., "I noticed that . . . ," "I felt. . . ."). Avoid writing in ways that distance yourself from your direct experience.

- **Your writing will create new understandings.** One of the exciting things that participants discover doing SP/SR is that writing is not the product of thinking; writing *is* thinking. Writing is a core part of the reflective process. Through writing, participants often find themselves able to recall new elements of an experience, develop new perspectives, and reach new understandings.

- **Write honestly because you are not writing for an audience.** Until you share your reflections in the public space, all your reflections in the workbook are just for you. You should aim for them to be as honest and authentic as you can make them in order to gain the most from the experience.

Taking Care of Yourself

- **Reflect on your needs**. If you do not want to engage with a particular task or a particular module (e.g., you are under severe stress and doing the exercise might add to that stress), then we suggest that in its place, you use the time and space to reflect on what you need to do to take care of yourself.

- **Do not expect perfection, it is unattainable!** Many individuals find themselves starting to question their clinical skills or effectiveness as a therapist. Through being in the client role, they may become more aware of deficiencies that were previously outside of their awareness, and may realize that they have not been performing as well as they thought. The adjustment of standards and expectations is quite a normal process when doing SP/SR, and usually settles down over the course of a program. It is always worth bearing in mind that the ideal therapist does not exist; we are all in the process of learning!

Building Your Reflective Capacity

Preparation

- Plan regular times for reflection.
- Be prepared for varied and strong emotional reactions.
- Be prepared for times of ambivalence.
- Plan to maintain continuity with SP/SR after breaks such as vacations or holidays.
- Find a safe place to keep the workbook and your written reflections.

The Process of Reflection

- Find a time and place where you will not be disturbed or distracted.
- Use an exercise such as a mindfulness meditation to transition from self-practice to the task of reflecting.
- Use strategies such as imagery and focusing on bodily sensation to enhance your recall of specific situations, and make you more aware of your thoughts and emotions.
- Do not censor your thoughts.
- Try and notice the unexpected.
- Notice whether you are reflecting or ruminating.
- Remain compassionate toward yourself.
- Use SP/SR to address self-critical thoughts.
- Reflection can happen in stages; revisiting previous reflections can be helpful.
- Ask yourself questions as you reflect on your experiences.
- Try and link the personal and the professional.

Self-Reflective Writing

- Use the first-person "I" for writing.
- Writing is a core part of the reflective process; the process of writing creates new understandings.
- Write honestly and remember that you are not writing for an audience.

Taking Care of Yourself

- Reflect on your needs, especially when you are feeling stressed.
- Do not expect perfection, it is unattainable! We are all learners.

The Three Therapist Examples: Shelly, Jayashri, and David

Throughout the workbook we will be referring to our three "representative" therapists, Shelly, Jayashri, and David. All the modules contain examples from one or more of them to illustrate how to use particular techniques. Shelly, Jayashri, and David are at different stages in their therapist development: Shelly is just starting out, Jayashri has just qualified, and David is an experienced therapist.

Shelly is doing her first training in CBT. She has been to some workshops and started consulting with clients. She has regular supervision. She has noticed that her mood is markedly affected by how her therapy and supervision sessions are going. Her tendency is to be highly self-critical of anything that she feels is "not quite right." For as long as she can remember, she has been a perfectionist. She worked hard, did very well at school, and was the pride of her family. At the undergraduate level, she felt stressed by her studies—rather unnecessarily so, she admits, as again she did very well in these.

She finds her CBT training challenging and stressful. In particular, lately she has found herself avoiding supervision sessions, or spending hours preparing for them. She feels very responsible for each client. If they are not improving, this distresses her. She feels she must be doing things wrong, and she should be doing things better. Her expectation is that both her clients and her supervisor are judging her as "not up to being a therapist."

As a therapist-in-training, Shelly has been advised to focus her SP/SR on a "therapist self" issue, rather than a "personal self" issue. She has chosen to work on her sense of incompetence as a therapist. When she starts to do SP/SR, she becomes very aware of how her views of herself are coloring her emotions and behavior.

Jayashri is a hardworking competent therapist who has just started out in independent clinical practice. Having transitioned into psychology from an earlier career in business, Jayashri has recently completed her clinical psychology training. She is now trying to consolidate all that she has learnt while coping with the increased demands of her new job and her recent marriage to Anish.

She finds it difficult to work with her clients' distressing emotions. When she reviews her sessions she has noticed that her approach can be overly cognitive in focus. Her supervisor has also commented on this issue. Jayashri is not sure why but has noticed that she feels very uncomfortable seeing clients in distress and finds herself rushing to do something to alleviate their distress, recognizing that this is often at the expense of helping them to understand what is occurring, and making longer term changes. This pattern is particularly pronounced when working with anxious clients.

Jayashri has recognized that her tendency to "try and make clients feel better" can result in inadvertently supporting the avoidance behaviors of her anxious clients. She has also noticed herself postponing therapy sessions where CBT interventions such as exposure and response prevention are indicated. She is keen to be the most effective therapist she can be and "knows theoretically" that she could help her clients more effectively by staying with, or even evoking, higher levels of emotion. However, she also believes that she should always make her clients feel better, and this makes witnessing distressing emotional expression very hard for her. To make things worse, she has at times become trapped in a cycle of self-criticism around her stuck patterns, which is lowering her mood during and after sessions. At these times, she can feel quite depressed.

Jayashri is very conscientious and highly motivated to make changes. As a newly qualified therapist, she can see specific elements of her therapy that she would like to improve. She has decided, like Shelly, to focus her SP/SR on her "therapist self." Her goals for the SP/SR workbook are (1) to understand the pattern that she keeps falling into, (2) to make significant changes to her ability to work with emotion in sessions, and (3) to become a better therapist.

David is in his mid-50s. He has worked for many years as a psychotherapist in private practice. His original training was as a transactional analyst, and over the years he has attended many different training workshops and is interested in a number of different psychotherapy models. He has recently secured a position in a counseling center focusing primarily on the treatment of clients who have a diagnosis of one of the anxiety disorders. The treatment of choice for the center is short-term CBT.

David feels confident in his ability to engage clients in the therapy process and considers himself quite competent when using the eclectic style of psychotherapy he has used over the years. In his new job, however, he feels somewhat pressured by the management to fit in with the service model. He believes that his long experience and breadth of knowledge is not really appreciated by his colleagues and he feels scrutinized, and sometimes judged by his much younger supervisor who is an accredited CBT therapist. This makes him anxious and sometimes angry.

David also recognizes that he often feels evaluated and negatively judged by other colleagues at work and by people he meets socially, particularly the friends of his partner, Karen. He realizes that this results in him making excuses and trying to get out of social events with Karen. This hurts her feelings and is starting to affect their relationship. David has dipped into CBT books and attended several short workshops on various aspects of CBT, but he has not completed a formal CBT training. He is interested in the CBT model but believes it to be somewhat superficial, and has doubts about short-term interventions. His supervisor has made the suggestion that an SP/SR workbook may be a useful way to learn more about CBT and its application. Having undergone personal therapy as part of his original training he is both intrigued by and skeptical of this idea, and has decided to give it a go. He recognizes that being anxious about what others think about him has been an issue that has dogged him throughout his life. He has therefore chosen to work on this problem from a personal rather than a professional perspective.

We hope that the examples of Shelly, Jayashri, and David in the modules will give you a feel for the ways in which the SP/SR exercises can be used.

CHAPTER 4

Guidance for SP/SR Facilitators

The creation of successful SP/SR programs has been among the most rewarding experiences that we have had as CBT trainers. Participants who benefit from SP/SR typically report a series of "aha" moments, gaining insight, knowledge, and skills in greater abundance than is usually afforded by standard training techniques. As a facilitator of SP/SR programs, there is a considerable sense of satisfaction derived from seeing participants really "get it."

This chapter has been written to support trainers and practitioners using *Experiencing CBT from the Inside Out* to facilitate SP/SR groups. These groups might be peer-led or trainer-led groups using the workbook for professional development; or trainer-led groups where the workbook is integrated with an existing university- or work-based CBT training program.

The present chapter is largely informed by the needs of SP/SR participants that we identified in Chapter 3, and should be read in conjunction with that chapter. If facilitating an SP/SR group is not part of your current agenda, you may still find this chapter of interest, but it is not essential to your participation in the *Experiencing CBT from the Inside Out* program.

The chapter is divided into four sections. The first section addresses the facilitator's role in an SP/SR program. The second section focuses on the needs of your SP/SR group. The third section covers guidelines for preparing your group for an SP/SR program; we highlight the central role of the program prospectus and pregroup meeting for preparing your group, and the importance of providing a strong rationale for SP/SR, reaching clearly agreed understandings of program requirements, and creating a feeling of safety with the process. In the fourth section, we suggest ways to "oil the wheels" of the SP/SR process during the rollout of the program, so that participants remain motivated and engaged and derive the greatest benefit.

The Role of the SP/SR Facilitator

We use the term "facilitator" rather than "trainer" advisedly in the context of running SP/SR programs. Facilitating an SP/SR program is different from teaching a "usual" CBT training program; it requires different skills.[2, 95] The trainer role in usual CBT programs is to develop CBT knowledge and skills through the use of lectures, readings, modeling, role plays, supervision, and feedback on performance; the focus is on the teaching and development of skills for use "out there."

In contrast, the focus of SP/SR is on the self; this may be the "therapist self" or the "personal self," but in either case SP/SR is liable to arouse anxieties, self-doubt, frustration, and on occasions a degree of distress. SP/SR programs last over a number of weeks and tend to make greater emotional demands on participants than usual CBT programs since the learning is from self-experiential exercises and self-reflection, rather than from an external source of expertise (a trainer or book). Thus, there is a rather greater need for trainers/facilitators to be sensitive to participants' individual needs and anxieties within an SP/SR context than within a usual CBT training program. A key role is to create a safe, smooth-running process, which anticipates and removes the barriers to participants' experiential learning.

The Role of the SP/SR Facilitator

- The SP/SR facilitator's role is different from the "usual" CBT trainer role.
- A collaborative relationship with the SP/SR participants is central.
- Key tasks include ensuring that:
  - Participants understand the rationale for SP/SR.
  - Are clear and comfortable with the course requirements (if applicable).
  - Feel safe with the process.
  - Are well engaged with the group process.

Central to the facilitator role is the collaborative relationship. Just as the collaborative relationship with clients is central to good cognitive-behavioral therapy, so too with SP/SR group members it is crucial to creating a well-functioning group. SP/SR is unlikely to work well if participants feel coerced; under such conditions, they are likely only to "go through the motions." Therefore, prior to the start of the program, the facilitator needs to ensure that participants understand and are engaged with the rationale for doing SP/SR; are clear about and comfortable with the course requirements; and feel safe.

Another important skill is creating conditions for effective group interaction in order to form a learning community, since the principal mode of learning is from each other's reflections rather than from an expert trainer.[17, 19] The role includes setting up a safe forum and keeping a watchful eye on the group process, contributing where appropriate and noticing if any participants appear to be struggling.

The remainder of this chapter expands on the facilitator's role, identifying key tools and processes for creating successful SP/SR programs.

Aligning the SP/SR Program with Participants' Competencies and Needs

As we have indicated, a wide range of participants at all levels of experience benefit from SP/SR. However, it is axiomatic that in creating an SP/SR program the facilitator should aim to closely align it to participants' competencies and needs.

For some people, SP/SR may be a daunting prospect because of its focus on the personal; others may view it as a "breath of fresh air." Some groups may be doing SP/SR as part of an introductory CBT training program; others may already be highly proficient in CBT. For some, SP/SR may be a compulsory part of an accredited program; others may have eagerly paid to participate. Some participants already have well-developed reflective skills; for others, reflection may be foreign territory. Some may work or study together; others may have little or no previous relationship. The facilitator's approach must necessarily be attuned to the group's needs. For instance, it is likely that participants for whom SP/SR is a compulsory part of their training program, or who have little experience of personal development work, may need rather more acculturation and acclimatization to SP/SR than participants who have voluntarily joined an SP/SR program.[2] For participants with less therapy experience or intrinsic motivation, preparatory information and discussion are likely to be particularly important.

Experiencing CBT from the Inside Out should therefore be used flexibly and tailored according to the group's experience and needs. As a general principle, the facilitator should aim to create a relatively homogenous group with a similar level of knowledge and skill; otherwise the coherence of the group is threatened and group members may find themselves challenged or frustrated by fellow group members.

Adjustments for different groups' needs can easily be made by changing the self-reflective questions at the end of each module.[16, 95] For instance, SP/SR for CBT supervisors can include reflective questions about the implications of the module for supervision to help participants fully integrate their experiences with their wider roles. Or if the SP/SR is integrated with an existing CBT training program that has a focus on CBT for depression, participants could be asked to draw out the implications of their experience of behavioral activation for their treatment of clients with depression. More advanced or specialized SP/SR programs might ask participants to identify and reflect on their assumptions about people from other cultural or ethnic groups, and the implications for their work with clients from these communities.

As we suggested in Chapter 3, adjustments can be made for the stage of development of the therapist. In general, for early career therapists (such as the example therapists in the modules, Shelly and Jayashri), the focus needs to be on turning declarative (factual) CBT knowledge into procedural skills-in-action. Here, confidence as a therapist might be an issue,[95] so it is usually advisable to focus the SP/SR program on the "therapist self" (e.g., "my lack of confidence when working with people with depression"). By contrast, a focus on "personal self" schema may be challenging but appropriate for more experienced CBT practitioners (such as David) to enhance therapist self-awareness, interpersonal skills, and reflective capacity.[15] These skills are particularly important when therapists are working with clients with complex problems who may challenge the therapist by triggering unexpected reactions.[93]

Participants vary considerably in their initial reflective skills. For some, self-reflection may be a familiar way of processing their world; for others it may be foreign territory. Some may reflect at length on their personal experience, but have difficulty in bridging to implications for CBT practice; while others may be avoidant of personal experience and self-reflection. To prepare participants, it is often helpful to explain the importance of reflection in therapist skill development[14, 27, 28, 30, 31, 35, 97]; to provide written examples of "useful reflection" from other groups; and during the program to highlight examples of particularly productive reflections from fellow group members. In the context of *Experiencing CBT from the Inside Out*, you should ensure that trainees' attention is drawn to the "Building Your Reflective Capacity" section of Chapter 3 (see pages 20–24).

Further ways in which SP/SR programs can be aligned with participants' needs are identified in the next section, "Preparation for SP/SR."

Aligning the SP/SR Program with Participants' Competencies and Needs

- The SP/SR program should be closely aligned to participants' competencies and to the needs of different training groups.
- It is preferable to have relatively homogenous groups in terms of skills and experience.
- Adjustments can be made for different SP/SR groups by:
  - Changing the self-reflective questions at the end of the modules.
  - Determining whether the focus of participants' SP/SR should be on their "therapist self" or "personal self."
  - Providing additional training and support to develop their reflective skills.

Preparation for SP/SR

The success or failure of an SP/SR program is in large measure determined by how well the facilitator negotiates the preparatory phase of an SP/SR program with the participants. In this section, we identify two key strategies, *preparing a program prospectus* and *holding a preprogram group meeting*, both of which can greatly enhance the potential for participant engagement and motivation.

Preparing a Program Prospectus and Holding a Preprogram Meeting

Any participant coming to an SP/SR program will want to know what he or she is committing to, particularly because of the personal nature of the material and the fact that it is taking place in a group context. With adequate forethought, preparing a clearly articulated program prospectus and holding a preprogram meeting can go a long way in alleviating fears and enhancing motivation to engage with the program.

The program prospectus should address some of the questions that will naturally occur to participants around safety, confidentiality, and the rationale for the program. This should be circulated to potential participants several weeks before the preprogram meeting. The preprogram meeting provides the opportunity to address concerns, answer questions, and tailor the program to meet participant needs. Facilitators should be as open as possible to changing elements of the procedure to ensure, in particular, that participants feel safe. Adequate time should be given for the preprogram meeting; we would suggest at least 2 hours. For some groups, particularly where SP/SR is a compulsory program requirement (e.g., for a university degree), a second meeting may be needed.

The prospectus and preprogram meeting should (1) provide a strong rationale for SP/SR, (2) create clear and agreed-upon program requirements, and (3) promote a feeling of safety with the process. These three issues are discussed below.

Providing a Strong Rationale for SP/SR

Effective preparation for an SP/SR program necessarily involves providing a clear, motivating rationale for undertaking the program. The SP/SR program prospectus should make the case for SP/SR so as to create motivation and an expectation of benefit. The prospectus may include quotes from leading CBT therapists such as Aaron T. Beck,[4] Judith S. Beck,[5, 97] Cory F. Newman,[12] and Christine A. Padesky,[1] and should summarize key research findings. However, as we suggested in Chapter 3, we would also caution against providing too much specific detail about the research so as not to create biases and expectancies that may affect the quality of the SP/SR experience. As an alternative to the program prospectus, facilitators could suggest that participants read Chapters 1 and 3 of this workbook, together with the reflections of previous participants (e.g., the quotes at the beginning of this book). Either of these strategies should help to create positive expectations and appreciation of SP/SR's potential value.

Testimonies from people who have done previous SP/SR programs can be particularly powerful (see frontmatter at the start of the book)—even more so if SP/SR programs have already been held locally, and previous participants can attend the preprogram meeting. At the preprogram meeting, the facilitator (and previous participants) can discuss the research in more detail, as required, including the value of SP/SR for skill acquisition and refinement,[16, 17, 22] the importance of reflective practice as "the engine of lifelong learning,"[14] and the integrative function of SP/SR.[16]

Creating Clear and Agreed-Upon Program Requirements

The parameters of the preprogram meeting will be different for different groups, depending on whether the SP/SR program is being offered as a standalone professional development program, or whether it is part of a formal CBT training program. As we have previously indicated, as a general principle it is helpful to be as flexible in your approach as possible, as different groups have different needs.

You will need to create agreements about program expectations, commitments and contributions, safety and confidentiality issues (these are addressed in the next section), and, in the case of university programs, clear guidelines for assessment. The preprogram meeting needs to allow enough time for these agreements to be arrived at collaboratively.

In regard to commitments and contributions: If written reflections after each module are part of the process, then what are the requirements? Reflections after every module? Active participation in the discussion forum? Timing and deadlines for posting reflections? Length and/or quality of reflections? What happens if "life gets in the way"?

Another issue is the time needed to complete each module. Facilitators need to allocate sufficient time for SP/SR. The combination of self-practice, personal self-reflection, and deciding which parts of the personal reflection should be made public (e.g., in a discussion forum) usually takes between 2 and 3 hours per module, sometimes more for participants who derive a lot of benefit. SP/SR should not be seen as "a little extra." There needs to be a realistic discussion about time allocation to each module. Clearly, allotting 1 week per module means that the SP/SR can fit closer to a semester structure. However, our experience suggests that some self-practice tasks—especially those in Part II of *Experiencing CBT from the Inside Out*—may be more effectively implemented over a period of 2 to 3 weeks. Facilitators should consider what aspects of the program to offer over what period of time. In some contexts, *Experiencing CBT from the Inside Out* may have greater benefit when offered over 24 weeks, or two semesters.

If SP/SR is included as part of a formally assessed CBT training program, then some other factors need to be considered. For instance, it makes sense to closely align the SP/SR program to the course curriculum. One pedagogically and time-effective way to implement SP/SR is for trainees to self-practice a technique shortly after that technique has been introduced through reading and workshops. For example, providing teaching on CBT formulation during the early stages of a program can lead smoothly on to the trainee applying his or her newly learnt formulation skills to his or her own identified problem area. Matching the content in this way can help create the scaffolding for effective learning.

A further issue for formally assessed CBT programs is that some form of assessment of the SP/SR component may be required. There is currently limited evidence regarding the evaluation of SP/SR reflections. The value of rating the quality of reflections for assessment purposes is questionable, and would need to be handled carefully due to the potential for creating demand characteristics around the content or creating increased anxiety in the participants. At this point possibly a safer alternative is to use an assessment process based on other products of SP/SR such as the amount of participation in the discussion forum or the amount of public SP/SR contributions.

Creating a Feeling of Safety with the Process

Perhaps the most crucial aspect of preparation for an SP/SR program is the need to allay participants' fears and create a feeling of safety with the process. The thought of SP/SR can invoke considerable anxiety. Typically, participants have two main concerns: fear of exposure to fellow participants; and in some cases, fear of losing control by uncovering thoughts or feelings that they cannot handle. For example, one CBT trainee commented that she was "not wanting to delve too deeply because you don't have somebody there to pick up the pieces if something happens."

Providing a clear program prospectus, which addresses the process of SP/SR and holding a preprogram meeting are critically important for creating a feeling of safety with the process. Without these elements, program participation may be distinctly half-hearted. The most important function of the preprogram meeting is to give full voice to trainees' concerns (ask something like: "What concerns do you have about the process from what you have heard or read to date?"); then follow up by eliciting ideas for addressing these concerns. Typically, participants will provide suggestions to address confidentiality and security issues, and the group will reach agreements around anonymity and confidentiality. These agreements should be recorded and circulated.

As facilitator of the meeting, you should ensure that everyone has a chance to raise his or her concerns and have them addressed. It is also important to be flexible, as some groups might want rigid boundaries around anonymity, while other groups may actually prefer to use their real names in their reflections.

One crucial element to emphasize in the preprogram prospectus and at the meeting itself is the distinction between *content* and *process*, and between *private reflection* and *public reflection*. As one participant reflected: "I need to be in control of what I'm spilling out. You know it totally has to be up to me what I'm writing and what I'm saying and by having an opportunity to write down and proofread it to see that everything is fine, everything is safe." Private SP/SR reflections should necessarily focus on personal experiential content ("I felt . . . my body . . . my images, my thoughts were . . . my reaction, and then my behavior . . . !"). However public reflections on the discussion forum should focus on process, not content (e.g., "I found it much more difficult to set up a behavioral experiment than I would have imagined. I found myself getting anxious, which seemed to interfere with my capacity to think how I could best test out my negative assumption"). Making the content/process distinction clear can allay fears about expectations and exposure.

Participants at the preprogram meeting may be reluctant to raise concerns about losing control in front of their peers, so it is often appropriate for the facilitator to do so.

As facilitator, you could say something like: "It is common for participants to feel discomfort at various times in an SP/SR program. This is normal, and usually quite tolerable. However, at times an issue can catch participants by surprise and arouse unexpectedly high emotion and distress. While rare, it can occur, so everyone on the program should have a Personal Safeguard Strategy,[3, 16] a graded series of steps to gain support from others in the event of serious distress" (see Chapter 3, pages 19–20, for an example of a Personal Safeguard Strategy). At the meeting, it is also helpful to reemphasize that, for the SP/SR program, trainees should choose a problem that is at a moderate to high level of emotional intensity *but* is not likely to be excessive or to cause major distress (see Chapter 3 for further advice about choosing the challenging problem).

The choice to remain anonymous or to use their own names in reflections should be up to the group members, and should be a group decision. Some groups choose to remain anonymous. However, on those occasions in which groups have chosen to use their own names, participants have reported the added benefit that the experience seems closer to the client experience in terms of vulnerability and self-disclosure. As one participant noted: "I do have a tendency to hide my insecurities, but funnily enough no one seems to have recoiled in horror as yet. It definitely highlights for me how difficult it must be for patients to do this, and we're not even sharing the content!"

Finally, the meeting should address your own role as facilitator and your relationship to the group. How will you act in the role of forum moderator? Will you contribute to the discussion forum, and if so, how? Do you have a dual relationship to the group (e.g., as facilitator and program assessor)? Might this interfere with the group process? How could it be addressed? Open discussion and agreements around these and other relevant issues will enhance participant confidence in the process and is likely to enhance the quality of contributions.

Preparation for SP/SR

- The SP/SR program prospectus and preprogram meeting are both key strategies to enhance participant engagement and motivation for SP/SR.

- The prospectus and preprogram meeting should (1) provide a strong rationale for SP/SR, (2) create clear and agreed-upon program requirements, and (3) promote a feeling of safety with the process.

- A strong rationale for SP/SR can be created through the views of leading CBT experts, SP/SR research findings, and the positive experiences of previous participants.

- Be clear about program requirements (e.g., level of contribution, deadlines, form of reflections, time to complete modules, assessments) and collaborate to negotiate agreements.

- Elicit all concerns around fear of exposure and suggestions to address these concerns. Reach agreements around confidentiality and security.

- Make clear the distinctions between content and process, and between private and public reflections.

- Raise the issue of "fear of losing control" if no one in the group does so.
- Ask participants to confirm that they have developed a Personal Safeguard Strategy.
- Emphasize that SP/SR participants should choose a challenging problem of mild to moderate emotional intensity (not major), and definitely not one that is liable to cause major distress.
- Address questions about your own role as facilitator, including the potential for dual relationships.

Oiling the Wheels of the SP/SR Program

Creating a Supportive and Enriching Group Process

SP/SR groups are learning communities. For many SP/SR trainees, the group is among the most enriching aspects of the program.[2, 17, 19] SP/SR groups usually meet in two contexts: online discussion forums and sometimes face-to-face group meetings. When groups work well, dialogue can flow and the process is enriching. The benefit of being part of a group doing SP/SR (as opposed to doing SP/SR alone) is that participants are frequently stimulated by each other's reflections to reflect more on their own experience and their implications for therapy. Their experience becomes normalized as they see that their colleagues are prone to the same kind of emotional reactions and similar difficulties in implementing CBT strategies. They start to recognize not only similarities but also differences from the experience of other group members, which can lead to a more nuanced understanding that CBT is not a "one-size-fits-all" approach.

Group-based SP/SR also provides the opportunity for modeling—for instance, trainees may better learn how to reflect by reading the reflections of their fellow trainees.[19] The group can also provide support during modules that are more personally difficult for some participants. Feedback has suggested that this support can play a crucial role in individuals completing an SP/SR program; during personally difficult modules the sense of cohesion and community can encourage participants to stay in the process or seek support from a fellow participant.

As previously indicated, the preprogram meeting is a vital cog in establishing group safety. It is vital that the group itself makes, and takes ownership of, the key decisions around process and safety. The meeting should arrive at clear agreements around confidentiality, content of postings, anonymity, Personal Safeguard Strategies, and an understanding of the role(s) of the facilitator. As previously mentioned, there are two ways that groups usually meet: online through posting reflections and group discussion, and in some groups, face-to-face. The group should determine when and how it meets—only online, or face-to-face as well?

Some participants are more used to online discussion forums than others. Instructions for access should be clear. It is helpful to demonstrate use of the forum at the preprogram meeting, and to provide hands-on coaching if required. Examples from previous discussion forums may be helpful, and the value of dialogue emphasized. It is preferable to use a discussion forum that can be accessed from work or home, on a PC or a phone/tablet. The forum should also be set up to send new postings to participants' e-mails to encourage them to log on and respond.

Beyond the initial preprogram meetings, SP/SR facilitators need to "oil the wheels" by encouraging, supporting and valuing participation, and responding to questions and comments in a timely way. They should keep an eye out for any personal or group issues that may be inhibiting participants, and troubleshoot any problems that might arise. They need to strike a balance between, on the one hand, "being present," perhaps adding commentary or questions where appropriate, and, on the other hand, remaining sufficiently in the background that the group is empowered to take the lead in learning from one another.

Face-to-face group meetings can add to the benefits of the forums, enabling more in-depth discussion about particular experiences or techniques.[3] These might happen on a regular basis where the SP/SR experience is closely integrated with an existing CBT program. In stand-alone SP/SR programs, group meetings might happen two to four times over the 12 modules. Our experience is that group meetings help further to "oil the wheels." However, they are not always practical if participants do not live close by, and sometimes they are not wanted by the group even though participants may come from the same region or work in the same organization. For instance, we have found that some professional colleagues working in the same city may be comfortable with posting anonymous reflections online, but are reluctant to discuss their reflections face-to-face. As with other aspects of the program, any decision to have face-to-face group meetings should be endorsed by the group.

The facilitation of face-to-face groups and the facilitation of online discussion forums are both sophisticated skillsets in their own right, well beyond the scope of this chapter to discuss in detail. If prospective SP/SR facilitators need to develop these skills, they should seek out specialist resources and training programs.

Creating a Supportive and Enriching Group Process

- The group should determine when and how it meets—online only, or face-to-face as well.
- The group should make and own key decisions around process and safety.
- The online discussion forum needs to be easily accessible and user friendly, with coaching provided if required.
- "Oil the wheels" by encouraging, supporting, and valuing participation.
- Carefully monitor the group process and troubleshoot where necessary.
- Access specialist training and resources if you need to enhance your skills in facilitating online discussion forums and face-to-face groups.

Looking After Participants

Our research suggests that the upside of SP/SR is that the insights can be rewarding and exhilarating; however there is also a downside in that SP/SR makes considerably more emotional demands on the participant than conventional CBT training programs.[3, 18, 23] Concurrent stressful life events can take a major toll on the amount of personal resources available to give to SP/SR.[2] For some participants (e.g., university students), a "head-down, avoid emotion" approach to getting the job done is often the most favored coping strategy. However, effective engagement with SP/SR necessitates engagement with emotion, which conflicts with a "head-down, avoid emotion" approach and may produce shallow engagement. Lack of social support can also lead participants to disengage from SP/SR, and sometimes to drop out.

Facilitators of SP/SR programs have a duty of care. They should keep a watchful eye out to see if any participants appear to be struggling. At the preprogram meeting, it is helpful to set up procedures that enable the facilitator to contact participants to see if they are okay, or for participants to let the facilitator know that all is not well as part of their Personal Safeguard Strategy. Facilitators need to be "allowing." There are times when it may be inappropriate to do SP/SR, or it may need to be undertaken in a reduced way. You may want to discuss what a "reduced way" might look like at the preprogram meeting. A default option may be to reflect on the value of self-care at times of stress, or to "drop out" for one or two modules. If disengagement persists, you should contact the participant to determine their needs, and discuss options with them.

Within the context of a formal training program, it may also be appropriate to have an alternative pathway (e.g., delayed SP/SR or reflection on its inappropriateness at this time or an alternative module), if it is considered that SP/SR is contra-indicated at that stage. For participants who have the option to choose the timing of their program, emphasize the emotional and time demands of SP/SR as well as the obvious benefits prior to their final decision, then ask them to consider if now is the right time.

Looking After Participants

- Facilitators have a duty of care to participants; they should keep a watchful eye and ensure that participants have Personal Safeguard Strategies.
- As facilitator, be flexible and "allowing" if participants are unable to participate fully at some stages of the process.
- For formal programs (e.g., those that are university-based), consider whether there could be alternative pathways in the event that it is not the right time to do SP/SR.
- If participants can choose the timing of their program, point out the time and emotional demands so that they can make an informed choice about when to start.

Concluding Comments

We are confident that if you follow the steps in this chapter, SP/SR will add a new and rewarding dimension to your professional development and teaching, which will pay for itself many times over in terms of the feedback that you get from participants. However, the role of SP/SR facilitator differs in a number of ways from that of the conventional CBT trainer role. Some CBT trainers may not feel entirely comfortable at first with taking on the SP/SR facilitator role. This is understandable.

If you have such concerns, we suggest that you consider what it is that you need to take the initial step: more information about SP/SR training programs? More materials? More facilitation skills? Greater exposure to the SP/SR research? Your own personal experience of taking part in an SP/SR program? Once you have acquired the resources you need, check whether you are now ready to design and start a program. If you find that you still have some negative automatic thoughts and unhelpful assumptions about running an SP/SR program, this might provide the impetus for a behavioral experiment, or a further action plan.

In conclusion, we suggest that facilitating successful SP/SR groups is a skill worth developing both for you and for your trainees. Participants often experience repeated "penny-dropping insights" and "aha" moments. This is exciting and rewarding both for the participants themselves and for the facilitators. Furthermore, it is not only participants who experience a deeper sense of knowing CBT. In our roles as facilitators, we have been privileged to bear witness to the reflections of participants. In turn, these have deepened our own understandings of the therapeutic process and enriched our skills as therapists, supervisors, and trainers.

PART I

Identifying and Understanding
Unhelpful (Old) Ways of Being

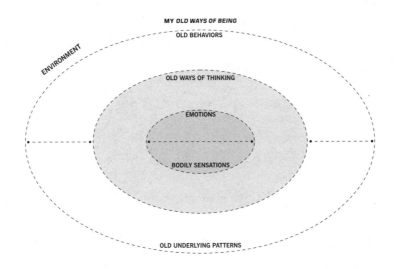

Identifying a Challenging Problem

> Completing this module has made me aware of how I perhaps skim over "outcome measures" seeing them sometimes as an "inconvenience" to those individuals who want to tell you their story and commence treatment. . . . Already my discussions around measures have changed. . . .
>
> —SP/SR participant

You are now almost ready to start your SP/SR program. Before doing so, you may want to refresh your memory of the three therapists, Shelly, Jayashri, and David, by revisiting their biographies at the end of Chapter 3. We will be using their experiences throughout the modules to illustrate the SP/SR exercises. You should also remember to establish a Personal Safeguard Strategy (see Chapter 3, pp. 19–20) prior to starting the program just in case you should become unexpectedly distressed at any time as you progress through the workbook.

The SP/SR workbook begins in a manner typical of CBT, by establishing some baseline measures so you can track your progress. This means creating an initial measure of your emotional state, identifying your "challenging problem," and constructing a purpose-built idiosyncratic measure with which you can track your progress as you work through the SP/SR exercises in the workbook.

EXERCISE. My Baseline Measures: PHQ-9 and GAD-7

The first task is to establish some objective baseline measures to track your progress as you engage with the workbook. To do this we suggest that you complete, score, and interpret two commonly used brief measures of depression and anxiety: the Patient Health Questionnaire–9 (PHQ-9) and the Generalized Anxiety Disorder seven item scale (GAD-7). These measures are included to provide you with a personal baseline and also to give you an experience, similar to that of clients, when first assessed. If you have a specific issue that you would like to address such as anger, low self-esteem, or lack of self-compassion, feel free to substitute your own baseline measure (see Module 1 notes in the Module Notes section at the end of the modules). You might like to search the Internet to see if there is an existing validated scale for your particular problem or emotion (e.g., worry, anger, self-compassion, difficulty tolerating uncertainty, perfectionism).

First, complete the PHQ-9, a standardized measure of low mood and depression: You can calculate your total score on the PHQ-9 by adding each item.

PHQ-9: PRE-SP/SR

Over the last 2 weeks, how often have you been bothered by the following problems?	Not at all	Several days	More than half the days	Nearly every day
1. Little interest or pleasure in doing things	0	1	2	3
2. Feeling down, depressed, or hopeless	0	1	2	3
3. Trouble falling or staying asleep, or sleeping too much	0	1	2	3
4. Feeling tired or having little energy	0	1	2	3
5. Poor appetite or overeating	0	1	2	3
6. Feeling bad about yourself—or that you are a failure or have let yourself or your family down	0	1	2	3
7. Trouble concentrating on things, such as reading the newspaper or watching television	0	1	2	3
8. Moving or speaking so slowly that other people could have noticed? Or the opposite—being so fidgety or restless that you have been moving around a lot more than usual	0	1	2	3
9. Thoughts that you would be better off dead or of hurting yourself in some way	0	1	2	3

0–4:	No indication of depression
5–9:	Indicative of mild depression
10–14:	Indicative of moderate depression
15–19:	Indicative of moderately severe depression
20–27:	Indicative of severe depression
	My score: _____

If you have rated yourself as being in the moderately severe to severely depressed range we would advise you to consider discussing your low mood with your supervisor, a friend, your doctor, or your therapist if you are currently receiving therapy. As we said in Chapter 3, you may need to decide whether this is the right time to engage in SP/SR. It is important to take care of yourself.

Now take a few minutes and complete the GAD-7, a measure of general anxiety. You can calculate your total score on the GAD-7 by adding each item.

GAD-7: PRE-SP/SR

Over the last 2 weeks, how often have you been bothered by the following problems?	Not at all	Several days	More than half the days	Nearly every day
1. Feeling nervous, anxious, or on edge	0	1	2	3
2. Not being able to stop or control worrying	0	1	2	3
3. Worrying too much about different things	0	1	2	3
4. Trouble relaxing	0	1	2	3
5. Being so restless that it is hard to sit still	0	1	2	3
6. Becoming easily annoyed or irritable	0	1	2	3
7. Feeling afraid as if something awful might happen	0	1	2	3

Copyright by Pfizer, Inc. Reprinted in *Experiencing CBT from the Inside Out: A Self-Practice/Self-Reflection Workbook for Therapists* by James Bennett-Levy, Richard Thwaites, Beverly Haarhoff, and Helen Perry (The Guilford Press, 2015). This form is free to duplicate and use. Purchasers of this book can download additional copies of this material from *www.guilford.com/bennett-levy-forms*.

Scores of:
0–4: No indication of anxiety
5–9: Indicative of mild anxiety
10–14: Indicative of moderate anxiety
15–21: Indicative of severe anxiety
My score: _____

✍️ **EXERCISE.** Identifying My Challenging Problem for the SP/SR Program

It is common as a therapist to feel self-conscious or to experience thoughts of self-doubt as you try out new skills and apply new knowledge (with varying degrees of success). Upsetting emotional reactions can occur in many different contexts in your work. Some examples might be: with a particular client, in supervision, or when you interact with peers or colleagues.

In this exercise, you will be exploring your experience as a therapist or in your personal life in order to identify a challenging problem to work on during the SP/SR program. We suggest the following:

1. Find a quiet space for yourself for this exercise.

2. Bring to mind some of the emotions and thoughts about yourself as a therapist that may worry or upset you—or about yourself as a person if you have decided to focus your SP/SR on your "personal self." (See Chapter 3 for guidelines around selecting a "therapist issue" or "personal issue.") We all have our own triggers. Can you identify situations where you think your emotional reaction is, or was, particularly strong or out of character? We all can run up against repeated problems in our work or find ourselves trapped in unhelpful ways of doing things, or behaving toward ourselves or others.

If you are focusing your SP/SR program on your "therapist self," think about specific situations when you have found yourself worrying or ruminating about your work, or feeling upset before, during, or after therapy sessions, lectures, or supervision. You may be upset when clients suddenly cancel appointments or do not arrive for sessions. Particular clients may challenge you, for instance, those with multiple social or lifestyle problems or with a set of values that clash with your own. You may find working with certain age groups makes you feel anxious, or you may see clients who reflect some of your own past or present issues such as bereavement or divorce.

You may dread (or even avoid) supervision or case presentations, wondering how you are doing in comparison to others, going over what you think others think of you, ruminating over comments that have been made, or double-guessing what your supervisor thinks about your work as a therapist. At these times you might, for example, find yourself feeling anxious, worried, upset, insecure, frustrated, or angry (emotions) and may be tense or tearful (bodily sensations), wondering how things will turn out, feeling scrutinized or criticized by others or what they might be thinking, or may be self-critical or doubt yourself (thoughts), and you might avoid certain kinds of referrals or react uncharacteristically (behaviors).

 EXAMPLE: Jayashri's Challenging Problem

Jayashri identified that she had a tendency to avoid addressing clients' emotion in her therapy sessions and this was limiting her effectiveness as a therapist. This tendency also exacerbated her self-critical side and this led to her feeling quite anxious and down.

All of the above can be experienced at work. You may, however, be experiencing strong emotional reactions in other contexts unrelated to work. If this is the case, you may prefer to use the SP/SR workbook to address a "personal issue" rather than a "therapist issue." You can use the same process as that described above.

EXAMPLE: David's Challenging Problem

David found himself feeling very anxious when preparing for supervision. He also felt anxious when he thought about attending his partner Karen's office Christmas party. His thoughts about each of these situations focused on the idea that other people might judge him as not quite measuring up. He decided his anxiety in personal situations was more problematic and therefore decided to focus on the personal rather than the professional.

3. In the box below list any challenging problems or situations that have occurred to you while reading the section above.

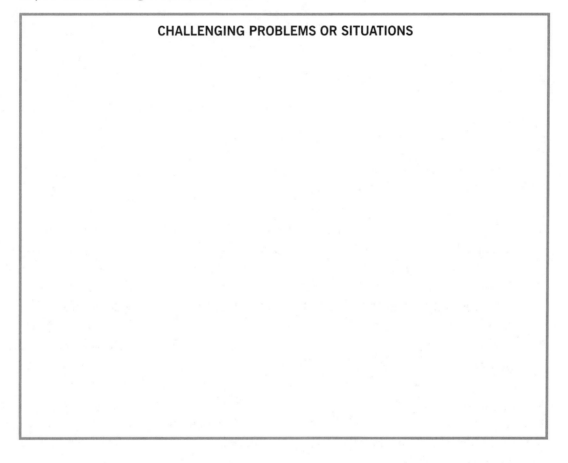

CHALLENGING PROBLEMS OR SITUATIONS

4. Looking at the situations you have identified, ask yourself which particular challenging problem you would like to focus on as you work through the SP/SR workbook. This should be a situation that causes you a moderate to high level of emotion, for example, *anxiety, frustration, anger,* or *distress* (an intensity rating between 50 and 80% would be ideal). It is probably a good idea to choose one of your more challenging or problematic areas. It also helps if this problem area occurs across quite a few situations. However, there are some exceptions. We strongly recommend that you do *not* choose a

problem related to an acute situation such as a significant bereavement, or relationship problem, or anything related to childhood trauma. Nor should you choose a problem that will cause you significant distress if it is not resolved by the end of the program.

5. Finalize your challenging problem and describe it in the box below. This can be a very simple description—for example, David wrote, "feeling anxious in social situations."

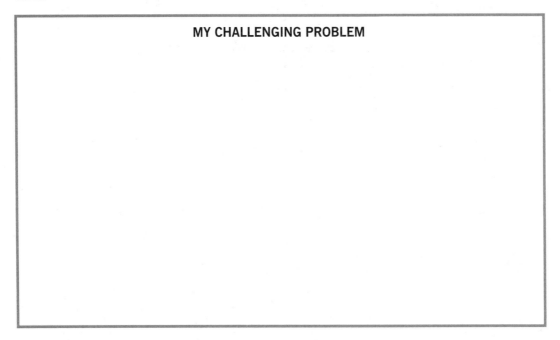

MY CHALLENGING PROBLEM

Developing a Personalized Measure: The Visual Analogue Scale

The next step is to develop and fine-tune a visual analogue scale (VAS) as your personal idiosyncratic measure. A VAS functions like a ruler or tape measure, and gives a number or rating to something measureable, generally the degree to which an identified problematic emotion, such as sadness or anger, is experienced. Using a VAS repeatedly over time is an easy way to keep track of fluctuation and change. When we set up a VAS we make it unidirectional in that it measures the amount of something, for example, sadness, where 0% is no sadness and 100% represents the most sadness ever experienced. When the VAS is introduced to clients for the first time, the client may be asked to give three different ratings to the targeted problematic emotion. First, he or she would be asked to describe a time when the emotion was experienced at its worst. This becomes a 100% rating. The next step would be to elicit an example of a 50% experience of the identified emotion, and finally, when the problematic emotion is absent, 0%. This process enables the client to perceive the way in which emotional states can fluctuate in terms of context. It also creates anchor points to help the client notice or identify his or her emotion in relative terms, encouraging more accurate rating.

 EXAMPLE: David's Visual Analogue Scale

David, after identifying his challenging problem as anxiety in social situations, set up his VAS in the following way. He remembered his highest level of anxiety, which he rated as 100%, as being experienced when he had to make a speech as best man at a close friend's wedding. When thinking about his problem at the start of the SP/SR workbook he rated his average level of anxiety in social situations at around 65% and noticed that he experienced no anxiety when he listened to music in the evenings.

David's Challenging Problem: *Anxiety in social situations*

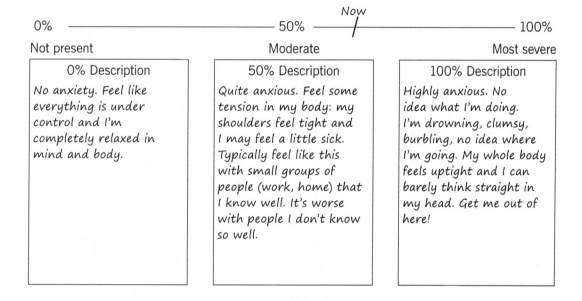

0% ———————————	50% —— *Now* / ———————	100%
Not present	Moderate	Most severe
0% Description	**50% Description**	**100% Description**
No anxiety. Feel like everything is under control and I'm completely relaxed in mind and body.	*Quite anxious. Feel some tension in my body: my shoulders feel tight and I may feel a little sick. Typically feel like this with small groups of people (work, home) that I know well. It's worse with people I don't know so well.*	*Highly anxious. No idea what I'm doing. I'm drowning, clumsy, burbling, no idea where I'm going. My whole body feels uptight and I can barely think straight in my head. Get me out of here!*

As you see in the example above, the VAS ranges from 0% to 100%. In the example, David generated extreme verbal descriptions at 0% and 100% to give his scale anchor points. He has also generated a description for a 50% experience of anxiety in social situations. This will help him to rate his levels of anxiety over time and to notice any fluctuations or changes.

 EXERCISE. My Visual Analogue Scale

Now it's your turn to create your VAS. Describe your challenging problem, then complete the VAS for your problem, as David has done for his in the example above.

MY VISUAL ANALOGUE SCALE

My Challenging Problem:

0%	50%	100%
Not present	Moderate	Most severe

0% Description	50% Description	100% Description

From *Experiencing CBT from the Inside Out: A Self-Practice/Self-Reflection Workbook for Therapists* by James Bennett-Levy, Richard Thwaites, Beverly Haarhoff, and Helen Perry. Copyright 2015 by The Guilford Press. Permission to photocopy this form is granted to purchasers of this book for personal use only (see copyright page for details). Purchasers can download this material from *www.guilford.com/bennett-levy-forms*.

Self-Reflective Questions

Now that you have completed all the self-practice exercises in Module 1 it is time to reflect on the experience. Before beginning, you may like to remind yourself of the "Building Your Reflective Capacity" tips in Chapter 3 (page 24).

What is your immediate reaction to doing the self-practice exercises? Was it easy, difficult, or uncomfortable thinking about yourself in this way? Did you experience any particular emotions, bodily sensations, or thoughts while you were doing the exercises?

_____

_____

_____

_____

_____

_____

_____

_____

_____

_____

_____

_____

_____

What particularly stood out for you when considering your reaction to the first stages of the workbook, namely, identifying a problematic area in your life and setting up ways to measure your progress in exploring or tackling this?

_____

_____

_____

_____

_____

_____

_____

_____

_____

_____

_____

_____

After rating your levels of emotion and defining your problem, what are your thoughts about the first stages of measuring and exploring a client's presenting issues? Has your experience of this "from the inside" changed the way you might do this with your clients? If this is the case, how will you do things differently?

_____

_____

_____

_____

_____

_____

_____

_____

_____

_____

_____

Is there anything else you have noticed that you would like to keep reflecting on during the next week?

_____

_____

_____

_____

_____

_____

_____

_____

_____

Formulating the Problem
and Preparing for Change

Reflecting on strengths was difficult at first, I seemed to be my
own worst critic however once I had identified them others came
easier as I started to feel better about myself. It gave me a kind of
mental boost, and made my problem seem not so problematic.
                                                              —SP/SR participant

The aim of Module 2 is to help you discover more about your challenging problem
and to identify how you would like this problem to change. You will be developing a
situational formulation of the problem, using a recent specific situation that caused you
some difficulty. The situational formulation uses the classic five-part model developed
by Christine Padesky and Kathleen Mooney: thoughts, behavior, emotion, and bodily
sensations in the context of the environment. Although this type of formulation may
be familiar to you, it is often surprising what emerges when you focus in on a specific
situation and identify the thoughts and emotions that you had at the time. Formulating
the problem can often help us to understand what drives it and why it keeps recurring.

Beyond the initial situational formulation, the module expands into what may be
less familiar territory. First, you will be examining how your background and culture
may impact upon your challenging problem. Then you will be developing a "problem
statement" to clarify the precise nature of the difficulty and provide a cogent summary.
The aims of the formulation and the problem statement are to deepen your understanding
of your *Unhelpful (Old) Ways of Being*.

In the latter half of the module, you will be taking some initial steps toward the development of your *New Ways of Being*. Having identified some of your strengths, you will be developing an alternative, strengths-based formulation, in which you identify how you would approach a challenging situation from a position of strengths. The last exercises are goal-setting exercises, looking at goals, obstacles, and strategies. The approach may be slightly unfamiliar in the sense that we encourage you to use imagery to set your goals for the program.

Module 2 takes the longest time of the first 6 Modules (we suggest 2–3 hours). You may want to allocate 2 or 3 sessions to complete it.

Descriptive Formulation: The Five-Part Model

As outlined above, in CBT one of the ways to think about problematic situations is to look closely at the different aspects of a problem in terms of five interacting areas. This five-part model, illustrated in the figure below, is depicted diagrammatically in order to highlight the way in which the components interact with each other to perpetuate a problematic cycle. The large surrounding circle represents the "environment" and the small connecting circles identify the thoughts, emotions, behaviors, and bodily sensations experienced in the situation.

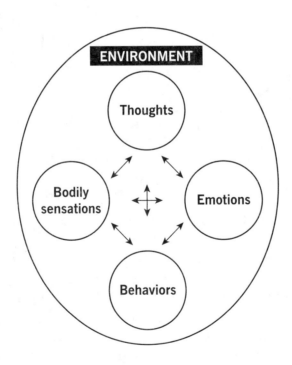

The five-part model.

Copyright 1986 by the Center for Cognitive Therapy; *www.padesky.com*. Reprinted by permission.

The "environment" includes the immediate triggering situation, along with a consideration of other background elements such as the person's developmental and social history, genetic makeup, spiritual/religious outlook, and cultural heritage. The double-headed arrows between the elements underline the interactive nature of the model. In this module, we focus mainly on the here-and-now, but bear in mind that a more detailed exploration of background factors can be important in CBT to give us a fuller understanding of the problem and its origins.

The Five-Part Model Summarized

1. **The environment:** In this context, the environment refers to two elements:
   a. The immediate triggering situation that prompts an unpleasant emotional reaction. Ask yourself: "Who was there?"; "Where did it happen?"; "What happened?" The trigger can also be a thought, an image, a bodily sensation, or a sensory stimulus such as a noise or smell. It is important to be *specific* in your choice of a situation.
   b. The past or present background influences such as history, genetic makeup, religion, spiritual outlook, and culture. We shall be further exploring the influence of culture in the next section.

2. **Thoughts (cognitions):** In this context, these are thoughts, images, or memories that pop into your mind in relation to the situation (automatic thoughts). As we shall see in Modules 4 and 5, if thoughts come in the form of questions, you will find it more helpful to change these to a statement in order to test them out (e.g., transform "What if I can't cope in my new job?" into "I'm not going to cope in my new job"; transform "What if I have a heart attack and die?" into "I think I'm going to have a heart attack and die").

3. **Emotions:** Emotions are often expressed as just one word (e.g., sad, angry, scared, anxious, or guilty).

4. **Behaviors:** Ask yourself, "What did I do?" or "What did I not do that I previously might have done or would like to have done?" Remember that avoiding something is also a behavioral response.

5. **Bodily sensations:** These refer to physiological responses such as heart rate; breathing patterns; aches or pains; dizziness; feeling sick; hot, or cold; or any other specific sensations or symptoms. Sometimes it can be difficult to identify a specific bodily sensation. Also look for general physical states such as fatigue or feeling keyed-up or tense.

EXERCISE. My Five-Part Formulation

Look at how David and Jayashri have constructed their formulations on pages 54–55. Using similar principles, complete the five-part diagram on page 56 to develop a situational formulation of your challenging problem. Remember specificity is important in identifying your thoughts, emotions, behaviors, and bodily sensations, so, if at all possible, find a *specific* recent situation where you felt a strong emotional response (an emotional reaction rated over 50%). This is invariably more useful than simply noting feelings and thoughts that might generally arise in this type of situation.

DAVID'S FIVE-PART FORMULATION

ENVIRONMENT

Immediate triggering situation
Accompanying Karen to her annual work Christmas party

Thoughts
I hate meeting new people
I have nothing to say to them
They think I am boring
They wonder what she sees in me

Bodily sensations
Tense shoulders
Rapid heart beat
Feeling sick

Emotions
Anxiety 80%
Sadness 60%

Behaviors
Standing alone at the bar
Drinking too much
Ask Karen repeatedly,
"When are we going home?"

Developmental history

Genetics and physical health

Culture

Spirituality and religion

JAYASHRI'S FIVE-PART FORMULATION

ENVIRONMENT

Immediate triggering situation
Client begins to cry in session

Developmental history

Genetics and physical health

Thoughts

Poor Jenny
It's terrible to see her so distressed
I shouldn't be upsetting her like this
I should be helping her to feel better
not worse

Bodily sensations

Tense
Increased heart rate
Heaviness in stomach

Emotions

Anxiety 70%
Confusion 80%
Disappointment 60%

Culture

Behaviors

Start to reassure client
that all will be well

Start discussing a less upsetting
item on the agenda

Spirituality and religion

MY FIVE-PART FORMULATION

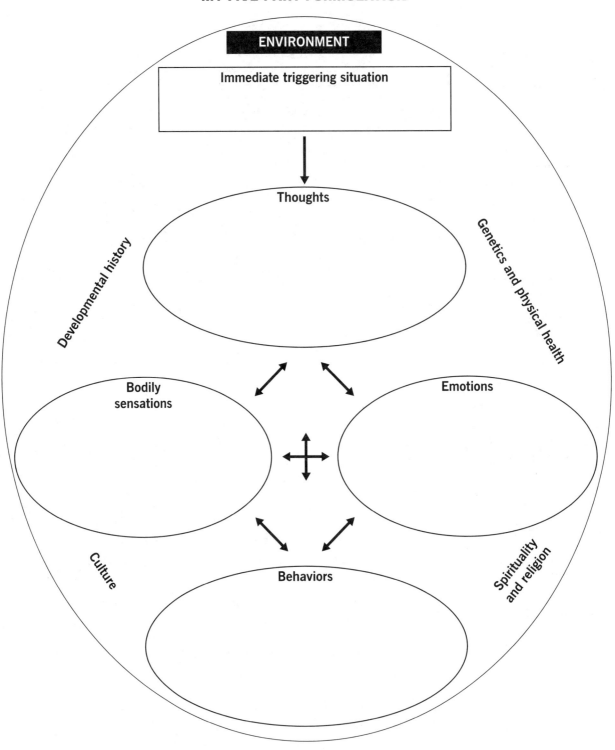

What About Culture?

You may also like to explore some of the influencing factors in the large enclosing "environment" circle of the model. One influencing factor that we often fail to consider is that of our culture. This is particularly the case if we belong to the dominant culture. In the West the dominant culture is sometimes described as Anglo/American. Individuals who belong to the dominant culture often do not consider that they have a specific cultural identity, believing that their worldview is the norm. We can think of this as "unacknowledged cultural bias." As our societies become increasingly multicultural, it is important to recognize the influence of our personal cultural biases, as these have the potential to impact upon the ways in which we experience individuals from other cultures and the ways in which they may experience us.

In contrast to individuals representing the dominant culture, culture is often experienced as very important by people who do not define themselves as belonging to the dominant culture. It has also been suggested that when we consider culture we should go beyond the obvious influences such as ethnicity and religion and consider other influences. Pamela Hays has introduced the "ADDRESSING" acronym to help us remember to do this. Identifying a personal cultural profile using the ADDRESSING approach can heighten our awareness of the possibility of unacknowledged cultural bias.

 EXAMPLE: The Summarized ADDRESSING Profiles of Shelly, Jayashri, and David

Have a look at the summarized ADDRESSING profiles of Shelly, Jayashri, and David.

SUMMARIZED ADDRESSING PROFILES OF SHELLY, JAYASHRI, AND DAVID

	Dimensions of Culture	Shelly	Jayashri	David
A	**Age and generational cohort:** The idea that different generations have particular characteristics, aspirations, interests, and lifestyles, which influence what they may attend to and what they think is important.	24 years Gen Y 1985–2004	36 years Gen X 1965–1984	57 years Baby boomer 1945–1964
D	**Developmental disability:** Groups of individuals who have been born with conditions such as deafness often express the view that they represent a particular cultural perspective and identity.	None		Mild dyslexia
D	**Disability acquired later in life:** Chronic physical or mental health conditions, injury, or accident.	None of any note		

R	**Religious and spiritual identity:** This is often more influential in cultures that do not identify as Western. Feelings about the importance of family, attitudes to women, and marriage can all be very influential.	Christian	Hindu	Agnostic
E	**Ethnic and racial identity:** Immigration is an ever-increasing phenomenon and many families are composed of several different ethnic combinations that influence how the family integrates into their new country. It is common that children born into migrant families may experience dual or multiple racial identities.	European	South Asian parents	European
S	**Socioeconomic status:** Defined by education, income, and occupation.	Professional/middle class		
S	**Sexual orientation:** Heterosexual, gay, lesbian, or bisexual.	Lesbian	Heterosexual	
I	**Indigenous heritage:** First Nation peoples (those who precede the settlers, colonizers, and immigrants).	None		
N	**National origin:** generally the country you were born in.	American		
G	**Gender:** Male, female, or intersex.	Female	Male	

Exploring Our Cultural Identity

In the form on pages 59–60 you will be creating an ADDRESSING profile for yourself. Pamela Hays suggests that we look at the categories in terms of the degree to which we represent the "dominant" Anglo/American cultural perspective. The more we "fit," the more likely we are to be: (1) unaware of our cultural bias and (2) have little experience of how it feels to belong to a "minority" cultural group. When filling in your ADDRESSING profile see if you can expand on the information.

 EXAMPLE: Jayashri's Cultural Identity Using the ADDRESSING Profile

Jayashri completed her ADDRESSING profile, which heightened her awareness of the subtle and not-so-subtle influences of her bicultural upbringing. Under the category "Ethnic and Racial Identity," she wrote:

> Both my parents were born in Hyderabad, India, and migrated to Silicon Valley, California, USA, in 1976. My dad is an engineer and my mom is a nurse. My family is Hindu. I was born in America but as a child we travelled frequently to India to visit the extended family. This does not happen so often now because

> my parents think it is no longer safe. My mom and dad were negatively affected by the attitudes of some people after 9/11 with Mom becoming quite depressed and withdrawn at that time. They often reminisce about the old days in Hyderabad but are pretty well settled in America although most of their friends have a similar background. I have married Anish, who also has Indian immigrant parents. We both feel pretty American. But we find we are much more aware of our cultural and physical differences from European Americans than we used to be. . . .

 EXERCISE. My Cultural Identity Using the ADDRESSING Profile

Complete the ADDRESSING form below. Expand on areas of particular relevance by using other sheets of paper, as Jayashri did in the example above, and identify those where you feel you represent the "dominant" Anglo/American cultural perspective.

MY CULTURAL IDENTITY USING THE ADDRESSING PROFILE

A	Age and generational cohort:
D	Developmental disability:
D	Disability acquired later in life:
R	Religious and spiritual identity:

E	Ethnic and racial identity:
S	Socioeconomic status:
S	Sexual orientation:
I	Indigenous heritage:
N	National origin:
G	Gender:

Referring back to their original five areas formulations, Shelly, Jayashri, and David considered that their cultural perspective or bias had influenced them in various ways. For example:

> **Shelly:** *Perfectionism and performance anxiety were part of my privileged upbringing where the individual must make her mark, make it happen, and do it excellently.*

> **Jayashri:** *The idea that it is shameful to show emotions publicly is something that my Indian parents have always emphasized. I wonder if this may be contributing to my immediate need to try and "make things better" for my clients?*

> **David:** *My experience of dyslexia may have contributed to my ideas that others might see me as not quite coming up to scratch. Being from a different generation to that of my partner and work colleagues may also be influencing my thoughts about myself as not quite fitting in and needing to prove myself.*

 EXERCISE. Adding Cultural Factors into My Formulation

How might your cultural background have influenced you in your life? Consider your original five-part formulation. Using the five-part diagram on page 62, add any cultural factors you think might be relevant for you.

MY CULTURALLY INFLUENCED FIVE-PART FORMULATION

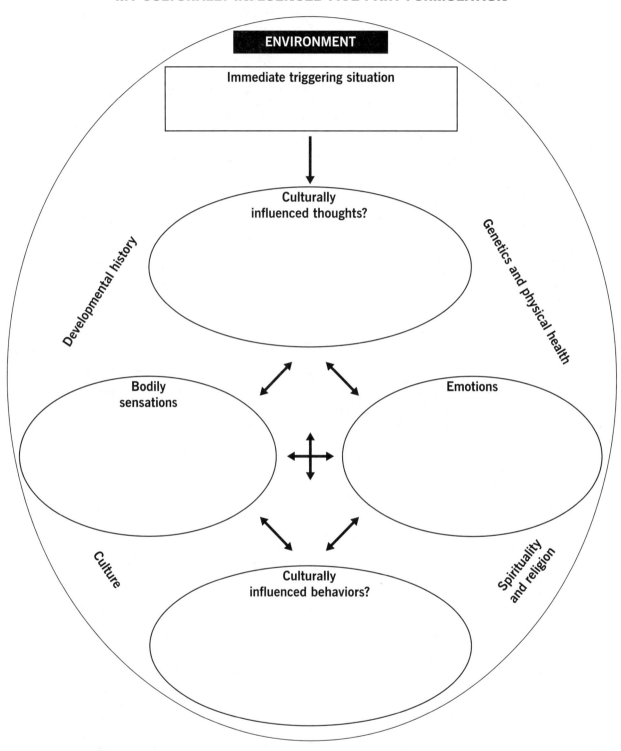

Developing a Problem Statement

Now that you have developed a five-part formulation of a recent work-based or personal experience, the next step is to develop a clear problem statement that reflects the CBT perspective that "one thing leads to another." The problem statement should (1) summarize the problem situation; (2) note the behavioral, cognitive, emotional, and physical components; and (3) identify the impact. You can see how this is done in Shelly's, Jayashri's, and David's examples below.

 EXAMPLE: Shelly's, Jayashri's, and David's Problem Statements

> **Shelly:** I avoid talking about my cases in group clinical supervision as I feel anxious and worried that I might be doing the wrong thing and others will think worse of me. This is leading to me receiving less and less feedback. And it causes me to feel less and less confident about what I'm doing.

> **Jayashri:** When I'm in sessions and start to see the client getting upset, I become very anxious and feel tense all over my body with a sick feeling in my stomach. I imagine the client getting stuck feeling distressed forever and I have a thought that I am a bad therapist and even a bad person. I then make attempts to avoid the potential upset e.g. move into less emotional content or try and make the client feel better.

> **David:** When I get invited to social events where I will be meeting new people, I imagine them wondering what Karen can be doing with such a boring old guy. I dread such situations and feel anxious and physically stressed, spending time thinking up excuses not to go or wondering what I can say to people.

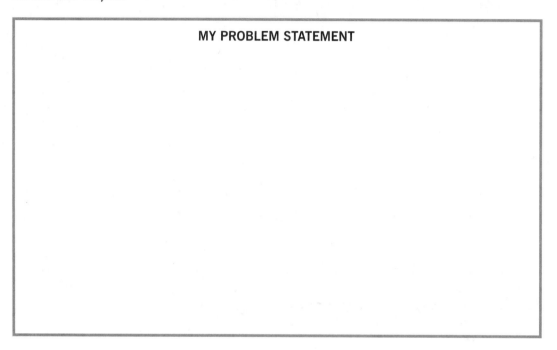 **EXERCISE.** My Problem Statement

Using your five-part formulation as a starting point, create your own problem state-ment in the box below. Express your formulation as a problem statement. Include the components of the problem: behavioral, physical, emotional, and cognitive factors; the upsetting situation that usually precedes the problem coming to the fore; and the impact all this has on you.

MY PROBLEM STATEMENT

Identifying Strengths

The previous exercises required you to formulate a situation where you experienced a negative emotion, and to develop a problem statement. Often we can spend more time noticing and worrying about what we did wrong rather than paying attention to situ-ations where we manage, cope well, or even shine! In the next exercises you will be exploring your experience as a therapist or person from a different perspective by iden-tifying and making a list of your strengths and creating a strengths-based formulation. Typically, the best place to look for strengths is in areas where you feel confident about yourself or in activities that you enjoy. These could be hobbies and interests or activities that are part of your daily routine such as exercise or cooking. Christine Padesky and Kathleen Mooney suggest that you view your search for strengths as a personal "talent search." What are your "X factors"? Strengths can refer to a variety of attributes such as good problem solving, sense of humor, intelligence, good manual or physical dexter-ity, and so forth. Consider your personal values and spiritual and cultural strengths.

Cultural strengths can be things like strong family ties, a helpful spiritual outlook, or a good work ethic.

 EXAMPLE: David's Identified Strengths

> *My strengths are a wacky sense of humor, a genuine interest in other people and what makes them tick and, through my experience as a psychologist, empathy and psychological insight.*

 EXERCISE. Identifying My Strengths

Record your strengths in the box below. If you find this difficult (as many people do), ask your friends or family members for some suggestions. You may be surprised at how many they may come up with!

MY STRENGTHS

Developing a Strengths-Based Formulation

To develop a strengths-based formulation, we need to make the strengths "real" to us by feeling them internally at a "heart" or "gut" level: the idea is to create an experiential awareness of how we experience these strengths emotionally, cognitively, and bodily. Next we cast our mind back to the problem situation that we formulated in our five-part model, retaining the felt sense of our strengths. Then we replay the same situation in our mind, imagining how we would have approached and experienced it if strengths-based memories and feelings were uppermost in our mind and body.

EXERCISE. My Strengths-Based Formulation

After reviewing David's strengths-based formulation on page 67, develop your own strengths-based formulation. Return to the problem situation, get the felt sense of strengths in body and mind, and imagine yourself experiencing the problem situation from that strengths position. See if you can reformulate it using the diagram on page 68 in a way that would reflect the strengths you have identified. What's happening in your body and emotions? What are your strengths-based thoughts and behaviors? Continue to add to the list as you identify more strengths in the coming weeks.

Tip: *Remember your strengths, as you will be focusing on these as you progress through the workbook.*

DAVID'S STRENGTHS-BASED FORMULATION

ENVIRONMENT

Immediate triggering situation

Accompanying Karen to her Christmas party

Developmental history

Genetics and physical health

Alternative strengths-based thoughts

I remember the times I have made my family and friends laugh.

There will be funny incidents at this party I can enjoy

I will take an interest in the people here as I do with clients

Alternative strengths-based bodily sensations

Feeling grounded and calm

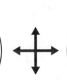

Alternative strengths-based emotions

Excited anticipation 60%

Culture

Spirituality and religion

Alternative strengths-based behaviors

Distract myself from rumination, focus on what others are saying and listen to them

Try and see the funny side of life

MY STRENGTHS-BASED FORMULATION

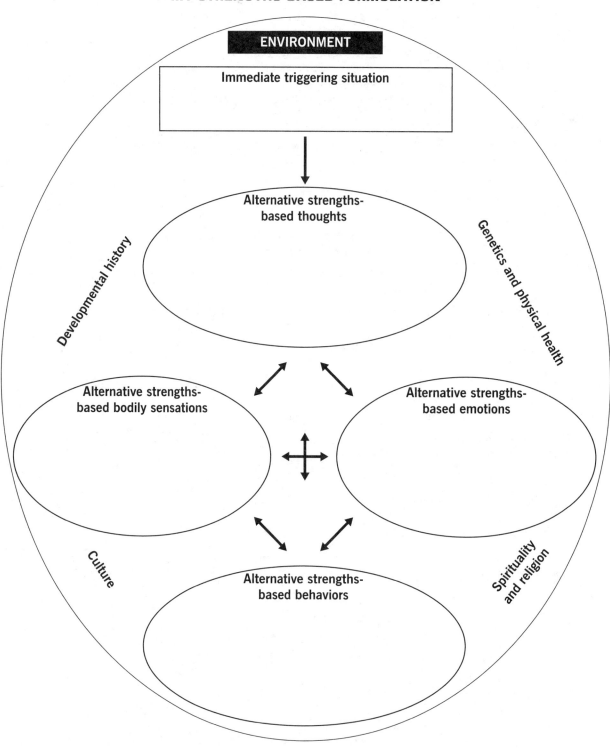

Setting Goals

With your five-part formulation, problem statement, and strengths in mind, it is time to create two or three goals, either therapist goals or personal goals, depending on whether you have chosen to focus on your "therapist self" or your "personal self."

Setting therapy goals can sometimes seem like rather a mechanical exercise. It need not be. We can use imagery to "bring to life" how we would like to be in the future. Imagined futures can help us to focus on concrete ways in which we would like our lives to be different. In the examples below, Jayashri and David used imagery to picture themselves at the end of the SP/SR program feeling confident and relaxed in situations that were currently problematic for them.

 EXAMPLE: Jayashri's Therapist Goals

1. To encourage a client who has a diagnosis of panic disorder to perform a panic induction experiment in the session.

2. When a client starts to appear upset, allow him (or her) to stay with the emotion rather than immediately trying to make him feel okay.

3. To be able to carry out Exposure and Response Prevention with a client to the point of optimal learning even if he or she becomes distressed.

 EXAMPLE: David's Personal Goals

1. To join Karen—without immediately making an excuse—when she asks me to accompany her to work-related social functions over the next 3 months.

2. To initiate a conversation with at least two strangers when I am next at a party.

 EXERCISE. Setting My Goals Using Imagery

In this imagery exercise, allow yourself several minutes of quiet, uninterrupted time. Read the instructions below, then close your eyes and experience yourself as if you have successfully completed the SP/SR program. Make notes about your experience in the box on page 70, and formulate your goals from what you have experienced.

You've reached the end of the SP/SR program. You have addressed your problem successfully. You have used your strengths. You have developed some different perspectives on the problem and have developed some new skills. How do you feel? Where do you notice that in your body? Imagine that you are looking at yourself through a video camera. What are you seeing yourself doing differently in the problem situation? Try and notice in detail what you are doing differently, how you are moving differently and feeling differently and thinking differently. Make some notes in the box below. Then translate these new behaviors, thoughts, bodily sensations, and feelings into goals.

Imagery notes:

My goals:

1.

2.

3.

SMARTening Goals

It is helpful to be able to monitor and measure progress toward our goals by creating goals that are SMART. SMART stands for **S**pecific, **M**easurable, **A**chievable, **R**elevant, and within a **T**ime frame.

EXERCISE. My SMART Goals

Develop one or two of your own SMART goals using the forms on pages 72–73. You can see how Jayashri has used the SMART form on page 71 to rewrite her initial goals according to the SMART principles.

One of Jayashri's initial goals had been "to encourage a client who has a diagnosis of panic disorder to perform a panic induction experiment in a session." After SMARTening this goal, she developed short-term (1 month), medium-term (4 months), and long-term (9 months) goals with clearly measureable outcomes.

Once you have reviewed Jayashri's SMART goals, rewrite your own using SMART principles.

JAYASHRI'S FIRST SMART GOAL

Goal [before SMARTening] *To encourage a client who has a diagnosis of panic disorder to perform a panic induction experiment in a session.*	**Achievable:** Are your goals achievable: just out of reach but not unrealistically so? *I feel confident that this goal is achievable if I get the support from my supervisor, which I feel confident I will.*
Specific: Are your goals specific? What are the dates, times, resources, etc., needed to achieve them? • *Discuss goal with supervisor.* • *Review diary.* • *In the first month, choose two clients with panic disorder. Conduct panic induction with both clients by the end of the month.* • *Continue with panic induction experiment for future clients.*	**Relevant:** Are your goals directly relevant to your life and getting things in order? What would you like to be able to do soon that will make a real difference? • *Relevant to effectiveness and confidence as a therapist.* • *Review literature regarding panic treatment. Improve confidence and competence by practicing induction in role-play and watching panic induction on demo DVD.*
Measurable: How will you measure progress with your goals and how will you know when you've reached them? • *Rate level of confidence in using panic induction before and after sessions.* • *Rate own levels of anxiety before and after sessions.* • *Review outcomes in terms of client feedback and progress with supervisor.* • *Record and watch sessions.*	**Within a Time frame:** By what date would you like to achieve your goals? Start with short-term goals. The addition of some medium- and long-term goals may be helpful as you progress. • *Short-term goal (1 month): To have performed two panic inductions by the end of the month.* • *Medium-term goal (4 months): To feel confident (8/10) in using panic induction experiments with clients with panic disorder.* • *To be doing panic induction experiments with at least 80% of my clients with panic disorder.* • *Long-term goal (9 months): Panic induction becomes a seamless part of my therapeutic repertoire.*

MY FIRST SMART GOAL

Goal [before SMARTening]	**Achievable:** Are your goals achievable: just out of reach but not unrealistically so?
Specific: Are your goals specific? What are the dates, times, resources, etc., needed to achieve them?	**Relevant:** Are your goals directly relevant to your life and getting things in order? What would you like to be able to do soon that will make a real difference?
Measurable: How will you measure progress with your goals and how will you know when you've reached them?	**Within a Time frame:** By what date would you like to achieve your goals? Start with short-term goals. The addition of some medium- and long-term goals may be helpful as you progress.

MY SECOND SMART GOAL

Goal [before SMARTening]	Achievable: Are your goals achievable: just out of reach but not unrealistically so?
Specific: Are your goals specific? What are the dates, times, resources, etc., needed to achieve them?	Relevant: Are your goals directly relevant to your life and getting things in order? What would you like to be able to do soon that will make a real difference?
Measurable: How will you measure progress with your goals and how will you know when you've reached them?	Within a Time frame: By what date would you like to achieve your goals? Start with short-term goals. The addition of some medium- and long-term goals may be helpful as you progress.

Strategies to Achieve Goals

Goal setting is important, but research suggests that goal setting has little impact without identifying and implementing strategies to achieve those goals along with strategies to address obstacles. What do you need to do to achieve these goals? How will you do this?

 EXAMPLE: Jayashri's Strategies to Achieve Her Goals

STRATEGIES TO ACHIEVE MY GOALS

What steps will I take to achieve my goals?

Tell my supervisor about my goals and put this on the supervision agenda as a standing item.

Diarize practice times for role plays with a colleague.

Track down resources such as a panic induction demo DVD.

Diarize a time to watch the DVD.

Before panic induction sessions, bring to mind times when I've done the experiment successfully with other clients.

What might get in the way (obstacles)?

The higher the intensity of the client's emotional reaction, the more difficult it is for me to push on with challenging exposure exercises.

How will I overcome these obstacles?

I'll make a cue card for myself listing the clear evidence for therapy interventions such as panic induction. I'll read this over several times before a session.

Recall my success experiences before sessions.

 EXERCISE. Strategies to Achieve My Goals

Use imagery to imagine in detail what steps you are going to take to achieve your goals. See yourself in specific situations making progress, confronting obstacles, and overcoming them. What are you doing? How are you going about it? What resources are you calling upon, internal or external?

STRATEGIES TO ACHIEVE MY GOALS

What steps will I take to achieve my goals?

What might get in the way (obstacles)?

How will I overcome these obstacles?

Self-Reflective Questions

How did you find the experience of applying the five-part model to yourself? What did you notice about the triggering situation, your thoughts, behaviors, bodily sensations, emotions, and the relationship between them? Were there any surprises?

_____

_____

_____

_____

_____

_____

_____

_____

_____

_____

_____

_____

_____

In this module you have used the five-part model in three different ways: to understand your problem (area of difficulty), to include aspects of your cultural identity, and to incorporate your strengths. How have these different approaches affected the way that you understand yourself and the problem you identified? Did any of them particularly resonate with you?

_____

_____

_____

_____

_____

_____

_____

_____

_____

_____

_____

_____

_____

Are there any ways in which doing the five-part model (including strengths) has changed the way you view yourself or the problem? If so, how?

_____

_____

_____

_____

_____

_____

_____

_____

_____

_____

_____

_____

_____

_____

Thinking about the ways in which you have formulated aspects of your area of difficulty using the five-part model, is there anything that you would like to introduce in your clinical practice? Do you anticipate any difficulty in doing this?

_____

_____

_____

_____

_____

_____

_____

_____

_____

_____

_____

_____

What did you make of doing a problem statement? Was this a useful exercise? If so, how might you incorporate it into your clinical practice?

_____

_____

_____

_____

_____

_____

_____

_____

_____

_____

_____

_____

_____

_____

Imagery was introduced into several of the exercises (e.g., strengths, goal setting, strategies). How did you experience this? Do you think it made a difference? If so, what kind of difference? From your knowledge of theory or research, what do you understand the value of imagery to be?

_____

_____

_____

_____

_____

_____

_____

_____

_____

_____

_____

_____

Describe your experience of self-reflection so far. Have you had any difficulties with the workbook? Is there anything you need to do to make things easier for yourself?

_____

_____

_____

_____

_____

_____

_____

_____

_____

_____

_____

_____

Is there anything that particularly stood out for you in this module that you would like to remember?

_____

_____

_____

_____

_____

_____

_____

_____

Using Behavioral Activation to Change Patterns of Behavior

. . . some refreshing findings for me personally and professionally. Linking this with client work I think I will be describing behavioral activation more as an "experiment" initially "let's find out and see" (as my own experience has proved that we really can't predict what will come out of it) and will certainly spend more time exploring clients experience of using [behavioral activation] as opposed to moving on too quickly to the next step.

—SP/SR participant

Exploring and changing patterns of behavior is one of the first things we might do with individuals who are depressed. Although you may not be depressed, behavioral activation is still a very useful exercise for managing uncomfortable mood states. We also often start therapy with behavioral interventions, such as behavioral activation, as our clients may often find them easier to understand and master. This is why behavioral activation appears as one of the first self-practice activities in the workbook.

It is hard to replicate the experience of being depressed. However, many of us, even if not depressed, struggle to do the things we would like to do or know would be good for us. Most of all we struggle with what we "have" to do.

Increasing behavioral activation and reducing avoidance can be a powerful way of improving the mood of our clients. However, behavioral activation strategies require care in the way that they are introduced. Many clients will have been told to "pull yourself together" or "just get on with things" so it becomes even more important that, when encouraging clients to engage in activity, we do this in a sensitive and understanding way—even better if our understanding comes from the inside out, from truly understanding how it feels to try and make such changes.

Many of our activities, behaviors, and patterns are performed automatically or out of habit and without awareness. If we want to be able to change these behaviors, then one of the first tasks is to increase awareness of these behavioral patterns and the impact that they can have on our mood. This is the purpose of the Activity and Mood Diary.

 EXAMPLE: Jayashri's Activity and Mood Diary

Jayashri completed the activity and mood diary on pages 84–85. As far as she was able, she did the diary at the time when the behavior occurred, or as soon after as she could, to maximize accuracy. She found that it increased her awareness of her patterns of behavior and she noticed various links between her behavior and her mood. Note that she chose three emotions to monitor and rate, depression, anxiety, and anger, because these were the emotions most highly related to her challenging problem. Below is Jayashri's activity and mood diary for the first day, Monday.

JAYASHRI'S ACTIVITY AND MOOD DIARY

	Day 1—Monday
7 A.M.	Got up and ate my breakfast, thinking about clients with complex problems I was seeing first thing. Depressed: 3 Anxious: 6
8 A.M.	Drove into work. Played some of my favorite CDs. Depressed: 2 Anxious: 4
9 A.M.	Saw client, it went well, and I felt like the week had got off to a good start. Depressed: 0 Anxious: 0
10 A.M.	Had meeting with my manager. Wanted to discuss going on some further training but didn't get round to mentioning it. Avoided bringing it up. Depressed: 4 Anxious: 2
11 A.M.	Had final session with client who had done really well. Depressed: 0 Anxious: 0
12 noon	Caught up on outstanding client notes and letters, annoyed that didn't have time for lunch. Depressed: 2 Anxious: 3 Angry: 2
1 P.M.	Session with client and had planned to do an in-session behavioral experiment. Client

	brought up new issue and I went along with this. Realized that we had both colluded to avoid the experiment. Depressed: 5 Anxious: 4 Angry at self: 3
2 P.M.	Session with new client. Went okay, still thinking about my previous session. Depressed: 4 Anxious: 3
3 P.M.	Client didn't turn up for session. Decided to pop out and buy some cookies to cheer myself up. Ended up eating half the box on the way back to the clinic. Depressed: 6 Anxious: 2
4 P.M.	Session with client, went okay though felt as if I was going through the motions slightly. Struggled to connect fully to what he was saying. Depressed: 5 Anxious: 2
5 P.M.	Had planned to go to the gym for a workout but felt so fed up I just wanted to get home. Drove straight home. Depressed: 5 Anxious: 0
6 P.M.	Made dinner, tried a new recipe, and it went well. Anish appreciated this too. Depressed: 3 Anxious: 0
7 P.M.	Rang Annie and caught up on how things were going. Discussed my bad day at work and she was having similar problems. Made plans for weekend. Depressed: 1 Anxious: 1
8. P.M.	Had a long hot bath reading a magazine. Depressed: 1 Anxious: 0
9 P.M.	Went to bed, decided not to stay up and watch the film with Anish. Depressed: 1 Anxious: 0

✍🏻 **EXERCISE.** My Activity and Mood Diary

Now it is your turn to record what you do over the next 4 days, together with the emotions you experience. Choose two to three emotions that have been troubling you in relation to your challenging problem and rate their intensity in the activity and mood diary on pages 84–85.

MY ACTIVITY AND MOOD DIARY

	Day 1	Day 2	Day 3	Day 4
7 A.M.				
8 A.M.				
9 A.M.				
10 A.M.				
11 A.M.				
12 noon				
1 P.M.				
2 P.M.				

84

3 P.M.			
4 P.M.			
5 P.M.			
6 P.M.			
7 P.M.			
8 P.M.			
9 P.M.			
10 P.M.			
11 P.M.			

✍️ **EXERCISE.** My Activity and Mood Diary Review

Looking at the last few days, are there any patterns you can see in your behavior or mood? Does your mood vary across the day or between days? Are there certain times of the day that are more difficult or certain activities that seem to be associated with a lower mood, increased anxiety, anger, or any other emotion? At the times when your mood felt low or you may have even felt depressed, what did you do to cope with this? Did this help in the short term? What about the long term?

MY ACTIVITY AND MOOD DIARY REVIEW

When we do exercises such as the activity and mood diary, it is easy for us (and our clients) to be hard on ourselves when we notice emotions and behaviors that are not helpful or if we are avoiding certain activities. What has been your attitude toward yourself? Have you been self-critical either of what you have done or what you have not done? What alternatives might there be? How would these serve your interests?

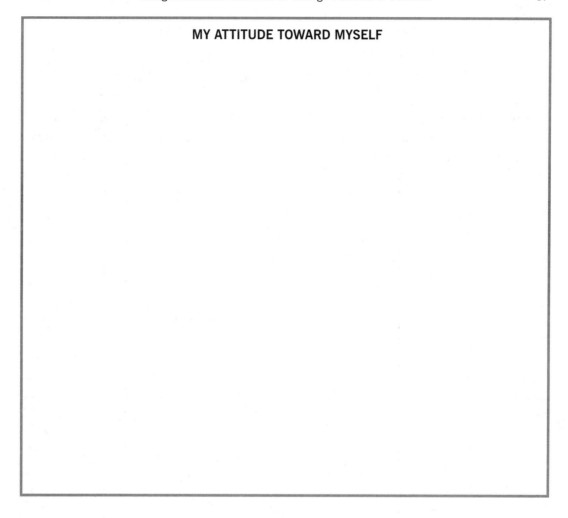

MY ATTITUDE TOWARD MYSELF

 EXAMPLE: Planning Alternative Pleasurable and Necessary Activities

The next step is to plan alternative behaviors or activities that might be more helpful. These can be scheduled at key times to replace less helpful behaviors or activities. For example:

Jayashri identified that when her mood was low in the evening she would often isolate herself by staying in the bath for hours or going to bed early. She realized that she was avoiding spending time with Anish some evenings, and yet on the occasions they decided to do something together, her mood usually improved greatly.

David found that when he was anxious in the evening, he would spend hours surfing the Internet and end up going to bed late no less anxious than when he started. As a result, he was frequently tired the next day. After completing the activity and mood diary, he made a decision to pay attention to his use of the Internet, reflect on his mood, and then do something more helpful such as telephoning a friend to discuss what was on his mind.

EXERCISE. Identifying Alternative Pleasurable and Necessary Activities

First, list some activities that are *usually* pleasurable and mood-enhancing: for example, going out with friends, going for a walk or swim, reading a book, going for a bike ride, going to a Zumba class, or the like.

Second, you will need to list activities that you have to do (or could "do with doing") but that might not be particularly pleasurable for you—for example, cleaning the house, paying bills, or changing your utilities provider. These are things you may have struggled to do, whether due to planning, motivation, time, lack of energy, habit, or avoidant tendencies. You might include activities that engage some of the qualities that you listed under strengths in Module 2.

PLEASURABLE AND NECESSARY ACTIVITIES

Activities That Are Usually Pleasurable

Activities That Are Necessary

EXERCISE. Creating a Hierarchy of Pleasurable and Necessary Activities

Having identified pleasurable and necessary activities that you are wanting to do over the next few days, the next step is to put them in order of difficulty from most difficult to easiest. Doing this will make the task of scheduling these activities into your week easier in the exercise which follows after.

CREATING A HIERARCHY OF PLEASURABLE AND NECESSARY ACTIVITIES

Most difficult

Medium difficulty

Easiest

EXERCISE. Scheduling Pleasurable and Necessary Activities

Using the diary format on page 91, schedule into your week some of the pleasurable and necessary activities that you have just identified. Identify specific times, people, and places (what, where, when, and with whom) and include a mix of things you think you might enjoy (but are not doing) and some that need doing. Plan for most of your time to be spent on the easiest activities; include a few items of medium difficulty and at least one or two of the most difficult, as identified in your hierarchy of pleasurable and necessary activities. It might be that you can identify specific times when doing these activities is likely to be more helpful than doing what you might usually or habitually do. For example, if you have found that you often lie on the couch after a hard day at work and that this makes your mood worse, plan an alternative activity, one that past experience has told you will be pleasurable or might provide a greater sense of achievement.

Carrying Out These Activities in the Next Week

Over the next 4 days, schedule these activities in your diary and record whether or not you did them. Also record your mood or emotion alongside the activity. Make an effort to do this in a spirit of openness and experimentation. When you are doing activities, it is a good idea to immerse yourself fully in them rather than evaluating the activities while you are doing them.

MY SCHEDULE OF PLEASURABLE AND NECESSARY ACTIVITIES

	Day 1	Day 2	Day 3	Day 4
Morning What? Where? Who? When?				
Afternoon What? Where? Who? When?				
Evening What? Where? Who? When?				

EXERCISE. Reviewing My Activities

After you have used the pleasurable and necessary activities log for 4 days, spend some time reflecting on your planned program. Then complete the box below.

REVIEWING MY ACTIVITIES

Did anything surprise you? Did you identify any particular patterns? Or successes, however small?

Comparing the last 4 days with the first 4 days when you only monitored your activity and mood, are there any differences?

Were there any times when you found that you could do something more helpful than you would have done in the past?

Self-Reflective Questions

Now that you have had an experience of planning and engaging in behavioral activation, it is useful to reflect on the experience and anything you can learn from this.

_____

_____

_____

_____

_____

_____

_____

_____

_____

_____

_____

_____

_____

_____

What did you notice about your experience of monitoring your activity and emotions? How easily were you able to notice any thoughts, bodily sensations, or feelings at the time? Or remember them later?

_____

_____

_____

_____

_____

_____

_____

_____

_____

_____

_____

_____

_____

Were you able to identify times where you responded to low mood or other difficult emotions with avoidance or unhelpful behaviors? If so, how did it feel to "spot" this?

_____

_____

_____

_____

_____

_____

_____

_____

_____

_____

_____

_____

_____

_____

What did you notice about the process of: (1) making a list of pleasurable activities or activities that you may have been avoiding and (2) planning changes in your behavior to do these activities? Were you able to follow through on your plans? If you were not able to, what barriers did you identify?

_____

_____

_____

_____

_____

_____

_____

_____

_____

_____

_____

_____

Was there anything that surprised you? How difficult was behavioral activation? What factors made it easier or harder? (How might this have been different if you were actually depressed?)

_____

_____

_____

_____

_____

_____

_____

_____

_____

_____

_____

_____

_____

Can you bring to mind one of your clients that you have struggled to "get moving"? Is there anything in this module that might explain why he or she may have struggled to engage or benefit?

_____

_____

_____

_____

_____

_____

_____

_____

_____

_____

_____

_____

_____

Can you think of at least one thing that you might do differently with clients in the future having experienced behavioral activation from the inside out?

_____

_____

_____

_____

_____

_____

_____

_____

_____

Have you learned anything about yourself through this module that you would want to remember?

_____

_____

_____

_____

_____

_____

_____

_____

_____

_____

Identifying Unhelpful Thinking
and Behavior

I was struck by how strong the automatic thoughts could be and how powerful the emotional reactions were. I was struck by the realization this was something I do so often with patients yet not with myself. I would have been very uncomfortable about anyone else reading this . . . yet I expect patients to do this freely for me as their therapist. I talk about how difficult they may be to spot and differentiate but not about the process of possibly feeling embarrassed or even ashamed about sharing them.

—SP/SR participant

All of us—clinicians and clients—can fall into patterns of thinking and behaving that maintain our unhelpful beliefs and behaviors and keep our problems going. In this module we start by focusing attention on some of the specific negative automatic thoughts that arise in challenging situations. The term "automatic thoughts" refers to the stream of thoughts and images that constantly run through our minds, mostly unnoticed. However, we can notice them when we give them attention, as you will have seen in Module 2.

Negative automatic thoughts (NATs) play a central role within the classical CBT model. They are understood to exert a strong influence on emotions and bodily sensations in the here-and-now, and play a central role in maintaining behavior. NATs are often idiosyncratic, laden with meanings or interpretations specific to that individual. These meanings are open to examination. NATs are often referred to as "unhelpful" thoughts to emphasize their role in problem maintenance. As CBT therapists, we are particularly interested in the *function* of these thoughts as well as the *content*. In Part II of the program, we will look at "deeper" levels of cognition (e.g., underlying assumptions) and at how we can create more helpful ways of thinking to embed the *New Ways of Being*.

Also within the present module, we turn our attention to identifying underlying *patterns* or *styles* of thought and behavior (e.g., avoidance, selective attention) that may subvert our best intentions in a range of situations. This "transdiagnostic" focus reflects an increasing recognition within CBT of the commonality of underlying patterns across diagnoses, and has led some writers to develop transdiagnostic approaches to assessment and treatment (see Chapter 2). In this context, we will be mapping out "maintenance cycles," another way of describing and formulating our problems. Maintenance cycles can powerfully illustrate how we get trapped into vicious cycles of unhelpful thinking and behavior that serve to maintain unhelpful mood states and behavioral patterns.

Identifying NATs

The aim of the first exercise is to identify and record your NATs in the problem situation on three or four occasions over the next few days. The instructions are the same each time, so they are only provided once.

One of the key principles for identifying NATs is to *Be Specific*. So the instruction here, and for our clients, is to bring to mind a recent, *specific* situation during which you experienced moderately intense emotions (40–90%) related to your area of difficulty; then to use a thought record (example below) to note the details. If you find it difficult to catch the emotions and thoughts, you might try using imagery to aid your recall: close your eyes and imagine the situation in as much detail as you can. In order to test the thoughts (as in Module 5), you should turn questions into statements. For example, you would change "Why am I so disorganized?" into "I am so disorganized." This statement is now testable, whereas the question was not.

It can also be useful to "unpack" the initial automatic thought in order to access more fundamental meanings. One way of doing this is to use the "downward-arrow" technique. The purpose of the downward-arrow technique is to access "hotter," deeper meanings of the automatic thought, which are often linked to strong emotion. Accessing strong emotion and "hot cognitions" is helpful for facilitating therapeutic change. With the downward-arrow technique we ask ourselves a series of questions to unpack the meaning of automatic thoughts, for example: "If this were true, what does it mean about me?"; "What does it say about me?"; "What might happen in the future?"; "What's the worst that might happen?" The example on page 100 demonstrates how downward-arrow questions can be used to access deeper meanings.

EXAMPLE: Jayashri's Use of the Downward-Arrow Technique

Situation

I noticed my mood dropping significantly during a supervision session when my supervisor and I watched a recording of one of my recent sessions. My supervisor made a comment about my therapeutic style, saying that I was a bit like a terrier and maybe I could slow down and demonstrate more empathy.

Initial thought	**Question to access deeper meanings or interpretations**
She thinks I'm a bad therapist.	
	If this were true, what would this say about me, my life, or my future?
I've been learning this for over a year and I don't think I'm ever going to be any good at this. I'll never be a good therapist.	
⇩	*If this were true, what would this say about me, my life, or my future?*
I will have to quit this job and look for something else. I don't know what else to do.	
⇩	*What would this say about me?*
I'm a failure, I'm a loser, and I never succeed at anything.	

Downward-arrow questions allowed Jayashri to understand how she was making predictions based on one comment by her supervisor. She knew that her emotional reaction to the initial comments was far greater than she had expected but the "downward-arrowing" helped her to understand exactly why. She was jumping to conclusions, predicting the future, and self-labeling. These are unhelpful thinking patterns that will be discussed later in this module. No wonder she felt so low by the time she got to the "bottom line." An important point here is that the downward-arrowing uncovered Jayashri's thinking pattern—it did not create it.

When using such questions with yourself or clients, it is important not to impose meanings that are not there or that do not ring true. Questioning is used in a subtle and speculative way to try and understand the meaning of the thoughts to the person. The process of doing this can evoke significant emotions, and whether using such questions with clients or yourself it can be important to acknowledge and stay with these emotions in an accepting and compassionate way. This is something that Jayashri found difficult, hence her supervisor's comment about her "terrier style." She tended to rush from thought to thought without acknowledging the depth of emotion that was evoked in the client. She also noticed that she followed a similar pattern when observing her own thoughts.

✍️ EXERCISE. My Thought Record

First look at how Jayashri has completed her thought record.

> One of Jayashri's initial goals was to try and understand the patterns that she falls into as a therapist, particularly her avoidance of clients' strong emotions. During the week, she had a few examples where she noticed herself slipping into a familiar pattern of behaving that was not helpful to the client. The completed thought record entry on page 102 details her experience in one of her sessions.

Over the next week, see if you are able to complete two thought records for two different situations, using the forms on pages 103–104.

JAYASHRI'S THOUGHT RECORD

Situation or trigger—where, when, what time, with whom, what was happening? The trigger may be an intrusive thought, a bodily sensation, a memory, a noise, or a reminder of some sort.	Emotions Each one can usually be expressed in one word but there may be several emotions. Rate their strength at the time (0–100%).	Thoughts, images, memories going through your mind at the time. Rate your belief in the thoughts at the time (0–100%). Unpack some of the meaning of the thoughts by using "downward-arrow" type questions to extract beliefs about self, the world, and others, for example, "What might it mean about me as a person, as a friend/mother etc.? What is so bad about that? What does it mean for my life and my future? If others knew, what would they think of me? What's the worst that might happen as a result?"
In session with a client with panic disorder. We had agreed to do a hyperventilation experiment that session and as the time came round to this I found myself feeling more and more tense.	Anxious (65%) Worried (70%) Annoyed at myself (85%)	I should do this hyperventilation session but I feel scared. (75%) I'm a bad therapist. (80%) I'm going to make the client feel worse or maybe even harm her. (70%)
Which thought seems to have been driving the most intense emotion? I'm a bad therapist.		

MY THOUGHT RECORD

Situation or trigger—where, when, what time, with whom, what was happening? The trigger may be an intrusive thought, a bodily sensation, a memory, a noise, or a reminder of some sort.	Emotions Each one can usually be expressed in one word but there may be several emotions. Rate their strength at the time (0–100%).	Thoughts, images, memories going through your mind at the time. Rate your belief in the thoughts at the time (0–100%). Unpack some of the meaning of the thoughts by using "downward-arrow" type questions to extract beliefs about self, the world, and others, for example, *"What might it mean about me as a person, as a friend/mother etc.? What is so bad about that? What does it mean for my life and my future? If others knew, what would they think of me? What's the worst that might happen as a result?"*	
Which thought seems to have been driving the most intense emotion?			

MY THOUGHT RECORD

Situation or trigger—where, when, what time, with whom, what was happening? The trigger may be an intrusive thought, a bodily sensation, a memory, a noise, or a reminder of some sort.	Emotions Each one can usually be expressed in one word but there may be several emotions. Rate their strength at the time (0–100%).	Thoughts, images, memories going through your mind at the time. Rate your belief in the thoughts at the time (0–100%). Unpack some of the meaning of the thoughts by using "downward-arrow" type questions to extract beliefs about self, the world, and others, for example, "What might it mean about me as a person, as a friend/mother etc.? What is so bad about that? What does it mean for my life and my future? If others knew, what would they think of me? What's the worst that might happen as a result?"
Which thought seems to have been driving the most intense emotion?		

Unhelpful Patterns and Processes of Thought and Behavior

The second part of the module focuses less upon the specific content and more upon the *patterns* of thought and behavior and the underlying *processes* that are maintaining your challenging problem. Researchers have identified a range of common patterns and processes such as escape, avoidance, and subtle safety behaviors that may strengthen unhelpful thoughts *and* prevent any new learning. The typical effect of these underlying patterns is to keep us "stuck."

In addressing unhelpful processes of thought and behavior, our task is to see if we can recognize any general patterns that are serving to perpetuate our problems. Five commonly identified unhelpful patterns, described below, are (1) cognitive biases, (2) selective attention, (3) avoidance or escape, (4) specific safety behaviors, and (5) unhelpful repetitive thinking.

Cognitive Biases

We are all prone to biases in the way we think, much like how a camera filter biases what is photographed through the lens. Cognitive biases include catastrophization, magnifying or minimizing, all-or-nothing thinking, personalization (blaming oneself), mind-reading, fortune telling, overgeneralizing, seeing emotions as facts, labeling, and disqualifying the positive. We all have "favorites" and often "specialize" in one or two of these at different times or in different mood states.

The box below describes the most common cognitive biases and provides examples of how these may function in real life.

Common Cognitive Biases

Catastrophization

Assuming the worst. Often people follow a chain of thinking that leads from a mildly negative or neutral piece of information to a worst-case scenario (this can be verbally or in the form of images). For example:

> My boss queried my expenses form, she must think I am trying to defraud the organization. I will be sacked. I will lose my professional registration and will be unemployable. I'll never work again and my wife will leave me. My children will be so ashamed.

Magnifying or Minimizing

Exaggerating the importance of a negative event and/or underestimating the importance of a positive event. For example:

> I actually managed to speak to some colleagues in my new job. They invited me on their Christmas night out. I wasn't very interesting when I talked to them and probably stuttered a bit. This means they'll never accept me as a colleague.

All-or-Nothing Thinking

Viewing things as either one thing or another without the ability to see the grey area in between. For example:

I know I'm a perfectionist but I don't want to change because either I'll ensure I do it perfectly all the time or I will end up doing it badly and messing things up.

Personalization (Blaming Oneself)

Assuming responsibility for an outcome that was actually a result of a range of factors. For example:

The work party was really dull and there was a weird atmosphere. It was my fault because I picked the restaurant. I really messed up everyone's evening.

Mind-Reading

Assuming that you know what other people are thinking which, at times, can be a very negative interpretation of what others are actually thinking. For example:

When my supervisor watched my tape and saw that I had missed an important response by the client, she would have thought I was an incompetent practitioner, maybe even that I should be struck off.

Fortune Telling

This is similar to mind-reading in that it involves an assumption that your belief is correct without you actually being in a position to know. In this case it refers to thinking that you know how things are going to turn out in the future. For example:

When I meet my new partner's parents, they won't like me and are bound to wonder why he is with me.

Overgeneralizing

Basing your belief about something (often yourself) on one small piece of perceived evidence. For example:

I can't even make a Sunday roast without burning it, I'll never be able to be a good therapist or a good father. I'm just terrible at everything I try to do.

Labeling

Making a global judgment about yourself or others based on one piece of information such as a one-time behavior. This is an extreme form of all-or-nothing thinking or generalization. For example:

I forgot my wife's birthday, I'm such a loser. I'm just a nasty and thoughtless person.

Disqualifying the Positive

Dismissing or underplaying the importance of a positive event or transforming its meaning. For example:

I know my colleague gave me a Christmas card for the first time this year but I think she is just being nice to me to get into my good books so she can ask me to cover for her next summer.

EXERCISE. My Cognitive Biases

Are any of these recognizable as a style of thinking that you are using with your problem? Note any biases, together with an example of each, if possible.

MY COGNITIVE BIASES

1.

2.

3.

Selective Attention

Are your problems being exacerbated by selectively attending to only one aspect of the situation? Where does your attention typically become focused when you are experiencing the problem—internally (e.g., on intense bodily sensations, or "failure memories") or externally (e.g., attending to danger cues rather than safety cues)? For example:

> David looked hard at people to try to pick up signs that they were bored with him. He interpreted someone yawning as meaning that he or she was bored rather than just tired.

> Jayashri ran a communication skills program for clients. She got great feedback from almost everyone, but found herself focusing on the one or two pieces of slightly negative feedback among the sea of praise and appreciation.

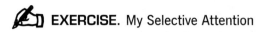 **EXERCISE.** My Selective Attention

---

MY SELECTIVE ATTENTION

Where is your attention focused (e.g., internal/external, cognitions/emotions/bodily sensations)?

What is the impact of selective attention on your experience of your problem?

Avoidance and Escape Behaviors

Are there things you are avoiding in relation to your identified problem? Are you avoiding doing certain things? Thinking about things? Or unpleasant emotions or sensations?

> Jayashri found herself avoiding situations that might lead to clients experiencing significant emotions—for example, doing a hyperventilation experiment. She also noticed that she was trying to escape from such situations when they occurred by shifting the session focus to something less emotional.

EXERCISE. My Avoidance and Escape Behaviors

MY AVOIDANCE AND ESCAPE BEHAVIORS

Note your avoidance or escape behaviors.

What is their impact?

Safety Behaviors

Safety behaviors are behaviors that we engage in to prevent an imagined bad outcome or catastrophe from happening. These behaviors actually prevent us from ever finding out what would have happened if we had not engaged in the behavior. While avoidance and escape can be seen as general safety behaviors, people often use specific *in situ* safety behaviors that can have a similar effect while appearing more subtle. For example, a client with panic disorder might think he is going to have a heart attack after he notices an accelerated heartbeat. He sits down (safety behavior) and does not have the feared heart attack but this outcome may simply strengthen his belief that it was sitting down that averted the catastrophe.

Shelly found herself overpreparing for all sessions and remained convinced that without the preparation the session would fail and her incompetence would be revealed to all.

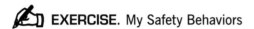 **EXERCISE.** My Safety Behaviors

---

MY SAFETY BEHAVIORS

Are there things you are doing to keep the worst from happening (e.g., in supervision, minimizing the problems being experienced with clients to avoid being criticized)? Note any specific safety behaviors below.

What is their impact?

Unhelpful Repetitive Thinking (Rumination, Worry, Obsessive Thinking)

Are you turning situations from the past over and over in your mind? Do you find yourself worrying about your problem more than is necessary? Are you being a bit obsessive about the problem or getting too wound up and detailed? How helpful is this?

> Jayashri found herself ruminating about her failure to stay with emotion in sessions. The thoughts went round and round in her head when she criticized herself. She tried to find answers, but remained lost in a cycle of worry and self-blame.

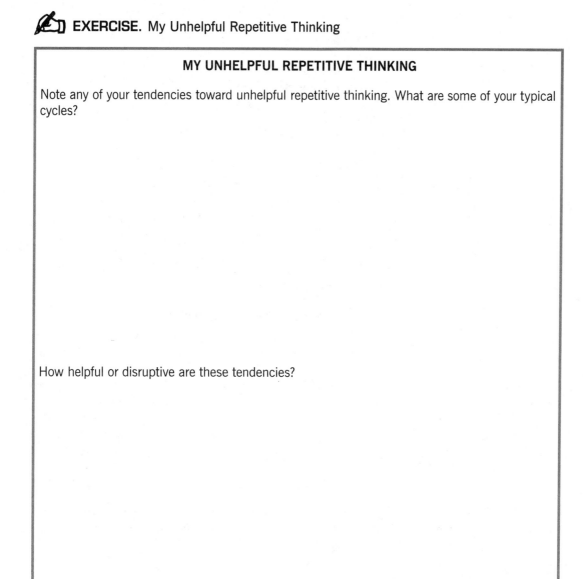 **EXERCISE.** My Unhelpful Repetitive Thinking

MY UNHELPFUL REPETITIVE THINKING

Note any of your tendencies toward unhelpful repetitive thinking. What are some of your typical cycles?

How helpful or disruptive are these tendencies?

Maintenance Cycles

One of the most effective ways to formulate clients' (or our own) problems in CBT is to pull together the elements we have discussed so far in this module and map them out into maintenance cycles. Maintenance cycles are pictorial depictions of how emotions, unhelpful behaviors, negative thoughts and beliefs, patterns of thinking (sustained by problems with information processing—e.g., cognitive biases), and bodily sensations feed into each other. Maintenance cycles take many forms and are often idiosyncratic to the client (or ourselves). They need to be individually constructed using the specific thoughts, emotions, and behaviors. They can then help us to plan interventions. You can see some examples below and on page 113.

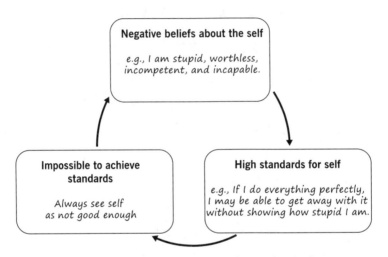

Example 1. Maintenance cycle for perfectionism.

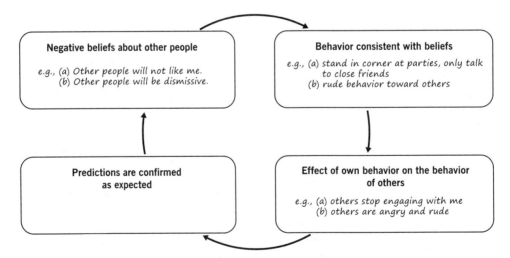

Example 2. Maintenance cycle for self-fulfilling prophecies.

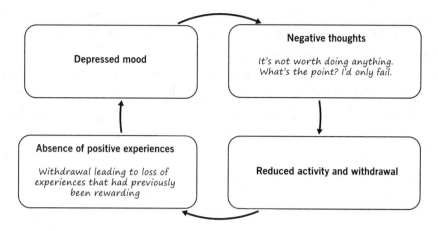

Example 3. Maintenance cycle for reduced activity and withdrawal.

EXAMPLE: Jayashri's Maintenance Cycle

Jayashri had identified that she was anxious about evoking emotion in sessions due to her belief that this would make her a "bad person" for upsetting her clients. However, she also knew that evoking emotion is often important and necessary in order to be effective. This conflict between her unhelpful and helpful belief made the situation worse, causing her to feel frustrated and annoyed at herself.

She mapped it out as below.

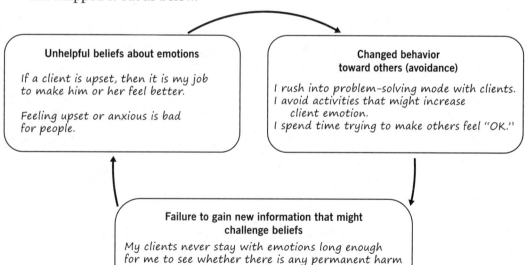

Jayashri's maintenance cycle.

In creating her maintenance cycle formulation, Jayashri began to realize that if she continued to behave in sessions as she was currently doing, there was no way that she could learn anything new or challenge her beliefs around client emotion.

It came as more of a surprise to realize that this pattern was not only limiting her therapeutic effectiveness but also was part of a wider pattern that had implications for her personal life too. It was a pattern that she exhibited with her friends, family, and partner.

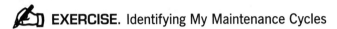 **EXERCISE.** Identifying My Maintenance Cycles

Map out one or more maintenance cycles that encapsulate your problem in the box on page 115.

MY MAINTENANCE CYCLES

Self-Reflective Questions

What did you notice about your experience of identifying negative automatic thoughts? How easy or difficult was it? How much did you believe the thoughts? Was there any difference in your level of belief at a "gut level" and at a "head level?"

_____

_____

_____

_____

_____

_____

_____

_____

_____

_____

_____

Having identified your own NATs, does this influence how you might work with clients to help them identify their NATs? How might you adjust or change your customary rationale? What do you think it might be important for them to know in advance (e.g., advance troubleshooting)?

_____

_____

_____

_____

_____

_____

_____

_____

_____

_____

_____

_____

_____

_____

Were you able to map out a personal maintenance cycle/s? Did you learn anything from this experience? Were there any surprises?

_____

_____

_____

_____

_____

_____

_____

_____

_____

_____

_____

_____

_____

Think about your current caseload and bring to mind one of the clients with whom you are having the most difficulty. How might the maintenance cycles that you have identified in yourself have an effect on your attitude and/or your behavior with this particular client?

_____

_____

_____

_____

_____

_____

_____

_____

_____

_____

_____

_____

What might be the best way to introduce the idea of maintenance cycles to your clients? What might be the best ways to develop them over the course of treatment?

_____

_____

_____

_____

_____

_____

_____

_____

_____

_____

_____

_____

_____

What are the key things you have learned during this module that you would like to remember?

_____

_____

_____

_____

_____

_____

_____

_____

_____

_____

_____

_____

_____

Using Cognitive Techniques to Modify Unhelpful Thinking and Behavior

> I do now see the problem differently after looking at the underlying processes. I can see how long I have responded in this way so it is understandable really. By confronting my avoidance and safety behaviors I think I will feel more at ease with helping clients to do the same.
>
> —SP/SR participant

In this module you will start to modify some of the thoughts, patterns, and processes of thinking and behaving that you have identified and mapped into maintenance cycles in Module 4. The module focuses on the use of Socratic questioning, the "cornerstone" of CBT, to explore your ideas and actions. We provide a number of examples of useful Socratic questions below. In some cases these questions can be used more or less as they are to test your thoughts. In other cases you may need to adapt the questions to the particular context of the thoughts or underlying processes that you are aiming to change.

Examples of Socratic Questions

- Am I focusing on one aspect only? What else could I focus on?
- Is there anything else I could include in my perspective of things—e.g., What might another person's view be and might it have any validity?
- What might a calm, compassionate, and rational friend, loved one, or someone I look up to say about this?
- What would I say to a friend who was in this situation?
- What am I overlooking here? Am I discounting information that contradicts this?

- Do I have strengths that I could use here that I have been ignoring?

- What are the costs and benefits of thinking this/avoiding this? How helpful is it? What would happen if I actually just did what I'm avoiding or faced the thoughts I've been avoiding? Would this be so bad? How bad?

- Is it helpful to keep thinking/worrying/ruminating about this? What could I do that would be more helpful?

- What resources or strengths do I have that could help me cope?

- How does doing _____ [safety behavior] actually prevent _____ [the worst] from happening? What would actually happen if I stopped doing this?

- Have I been jumping to conclusions that are not completely justified?

- How could I use what I have learned from previous similar experiences where things worked out to modify my view of this?

- Am I taking the blame for something that is not (entirely) my fault or over which I have no control?

- Can I see a short cut to an alternative view from my "biased" thought/s (simply by recognizing the cognitive bias I have been using)?

- What insights have I gleaned from mapping out my maintenance cycles that provide me with clues as to how or where I might intervene to address my problem?

Following Module 4, this module continues the focus on NATs and underlying patterns and processes. In the first half of the module, you will be devising or adapting Socratic questions to test out some of your NATs. In the second half of the module, Socratic questions are used to modify underlying patterns and processes.

Modifying Thought Content: Using Thought Records to Test NATs

One of the first tasks in this module is to practice modifying thought *content* using Socratic questions.

 EXERCISE. Using a Thought Record to Test NATs

In the box at the top of the form on page 123, identify a NAT related to your issue. This may be one of the NATs you identified in Module 4, or it may be another one. Use Socratic questions to test out the thought. Then see if you can complete a second thought record (on page 124) for a different thought during the week.

You can see how Jayashri has completed her thought record on page 122.

JAYASHRI'S THOUGHT RECORD TO TEST NATs

Write the thought to test here and rate the belief:

I'm a bad therapist. Belief: 80%

Associated emotion/mood and intensity (0–100%): Anxiety: 80% Guilt: 70%

What ideas or evidence led me to this conclusion?	What evidence does not support this?	Modified perspective/more balanced view	Rate emotion now (0–100%)
I'm not sure. Whenever I feel a client starting to get upset, I feel bad inside and start to judge myself. Hmm . . . . this isn't really evidence is it?	All the evidence shows that clients need to experience emotion to learn effectively. I know this rationally myself too.	(How much do I believe it: 0–100%?) I think I have been using emotion as evidence to support my thought without realizing it. I get good feedback from clients and my supervisor most of the time. This is starting to smell of "emotional reasoning." 20%	Anxiety: 40% Guilt: 20%
	On the rare occasions when I have encouraged clients to stay with their emotions, they have always told me that it was incredibly useful.		
	I get a fair bit of positive feedback from clients, even if I too easily dismiss it.		
	My supervisor thinks I'm pretty good on the whole.		

MY THOUGHT RECORD TO TEST NATs

Write the thought to test here and rate the belief:

Associated emotion/mood and intensity (0–100%):

What ideas or evidence led me to this conclusion?	What evidence does not support this?	Modified perspective/more balanced view (How much do I believe it: 0–100%?)	Rate emotion now (0–100%)

MY THOUGHT RECORD TO TEST NATs

Write the thought to test here and rate the belief:

Associated emotion/mood and intensity (0–100%):

What ideas or evidence led me to this conclusion?	What evidence does not support this?	Modified perspective/more balanced view (How much do I believe it: 0–100%?)	Rate emotion now (0–100%)

Addressing Problematic Underlying Patterns with Socratic Questioning

In the previous module you identified examples of patterns of thinking and behaving that were occurring in the context of your challenging problem; you also identified some maintenance cycles, which demonstrated how these patterns might be maintaining the problem. In this module we use Socratic questioning to explore these patterns further in order to change them.

What follow are examples of Shelly's thinking styles and patterns of behaving. These examples also include useful Socratic questions that she used to explore her underlying patterns. After the examples, you have the opportunity to return to your own previous examples (and/or add new ones), and use Socratic questioning—from the list at the start of the module or even better design your own—to start to change them.

Cognitive Biases

 EXAMPLE: Shelly's Cognitive Bias

> **My identified thought/process/bias:** *I am jumping to the conclusion that my client thinks I am useless because I am 20 years younger than him.*
>
> **The Socratic questions I have chosen:** *What is the evidence for this view? What am I basing it on? Is there an alternative explanation?*
>
> **My response:** *Instead of mind-reading, I could speak to the client about the comment he made (about my age) and see how we can address any concerns he may have (if any).*

 EXERCISE. My Cognitive Bias

> **My identified thought/process/bias:**
>
>
>
> **The Socratic questions I have chosen:**
>
>
>
> **My response:**

Selective Attention

 EXAMPLE: Shelly's Selective Attention

My identified thought/process/bias: *I am focusing on one comment he made in a session that I look like his daughter.*

The Socratic questions I have chosen: *What am I overlooking here? Am I discounting information that contradicts this?*

My response: *In the last two sessions, we have worked quite well together and his depression has improved. I am continuing to focus on his comment and its meaning when it does not seem to be an issue to him.*

**EXERCISE. My Selective Attention

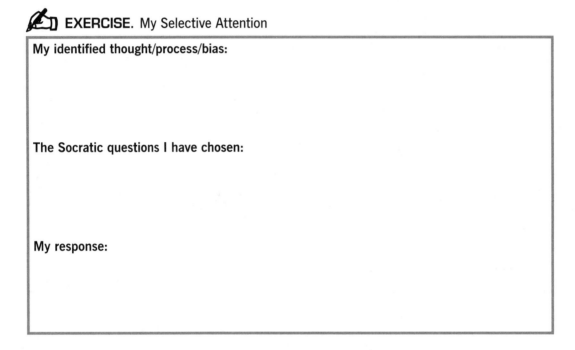

My identified thought/process/bias:

The Socratic questions I have chosen:

My response:

Avoidance or Escape (Cognitive or Behavioral)

 EXAMPLE: Shelly's Avoidance or Escape

My identified thought/process/bias: *I still find ways to avoid seeing older people. The older they are the more likely they are to comment on my age and the less likely I am to be able to help them.*

The Socratic questions I have chosen: *What effect does avoiding seeing older clients have on me and my anxiety about helping older clients? What price do I pay for this?*

My response: *It's just making it worse. I know deep down that it's become part of the problem rather than being a long-term solution. It's out of proportion too compared to my initial worry! I need to take a "risk" and see as many older people as possible.*

EXERCISE. My Avoidance or Escape

My identified thought/process/bias:

The Socratic questions I have chosen:

My response:

Specific Safety Behaviors

 EXAMPLE: Shelly's Specific Safety Behaviors

My identified thought/process/bias: *I find myself overpreparing for almost all of my sessions. If I don't spend extra time making sure all my sessions are planned in detail then I will be "found out."*

The Socratic questions I have chosen: *What information actually supports this idea that I'm not effective in my role? Have I had this thought before in other areas of my life?*

My response: *I'm confused as I can't think of any evidence that I'm not doing a good job. I feel like this whenever I get put to the test—undergraduate degree, hockey team, presenting at tutorials. I need to stop overpreparing so I can test whether I can do okay without spending hours and hours sweating beforehand.*

EXERCISE. My Specific Safety Behaviors

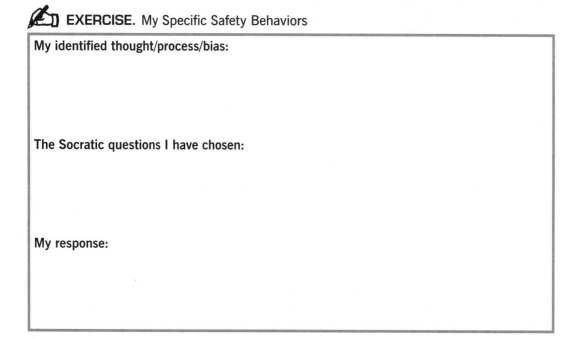

My identified thought/process/bias:

The Socratic questions I have chosen:

My response:

Unhelpful Repetitive Thinking (Rumination, Worry, Obsessive Thinking)

 EXAMPLE: Shelly's Unhelpful Repetitive Thinking

My identified thought/process/bias: *I am ruminating on this issue every day and have been for 3 weeks. Perhaps this is just a way of not facing my thoughts that I am never going to be an effective therapist.*

The Socratic questions I have chosen: *Is it helpful to keep thinking/worrying/ ruminating about this? What could I do that would be more helpful? Is the problem my incompetence, or my worry about my incompetence?*

My response: *I am going to focus on my therapy with him and do a thought record on my thought that I am a useless therapist.*

EXERCISE. My Unhelpful Repetitive Thinking

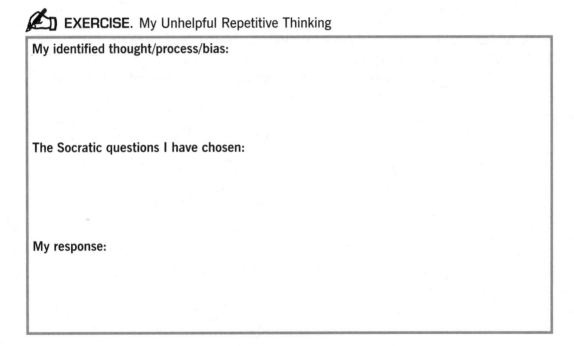

My identified thought/process/bias:

The Socratic questions I have chosen:

My response:

Problem Formulation Including Vulnerability Factors and Underlying Patterns

We can now create a formulation diagram that builds on earlier formulations (the five-part model and maintenance processes) by adding historical/vulnerability factors that are encapsulated in the question "What made me vulnerable in the first place?" When thinking about vulnerability factors, it may also be relevant to consider cultural and religious/spiritual influences as you did in your first problem formulation in Module 2. When considering "What have I got going for me?," it is pertinent to remember personal strengths that may also have a cultural and or religious/spiritual dimension.

 EXERCISE. My Problem Formulation, Including Vulnerability Factors, Underlying Patterns, and Strengths

See how Jayashri has completed her expanded formulation, including the vulnerability factors, triggers, and maintenance cycles, on page 131.

Now complete the expanded problem formulation diagram for yourself on page 132. Include your own vulnerability factors, strengths, maintenance cycles, and underlying patterns.

JAYASHRI'S PROBLEM FORMULATION, INCLUDING VULNERABILITY FACTORS AND UNDERLYING PATTERNS

What made me vulnerable in the first place?

A strong cultural message from my family that expressing emotion was shameful. Culture within family that females were responsible for caring and helping people feel better.

What triggered the problem?

Being in a session and knowing that I "should" be doing a task that will lead to the client feeling very distressed.

The Problem

Thoughts I'm a bad therapist.

Bodily sensations Tenseness in neck and back, whole body feels "uptight," sick in stomach.

Emotions Anxious, scared, uncomfortable.

Behaviors Collude with the client and focus on other tasks involving less emotion.

What maintains the problem? Include underlying patterns and processes driving your problematic thinking and behavior.

Catastrophizing! Having an image of a distressed person uncontrollably distressed and it not ending. Believing this to be true and thus increasing my anxiety.

Cognitive avoidance: Trying to shut such thoughts out instead of working through them and thereby maintaining a sense of on-going fear and discomfort.

Avoidance in session: Avoiding tasks that evoke or maintain clients' distress so that I have no chance to prove it is usually more helpful for the client's progress to stay with the distress and work through it.

What have I got going for me: Strengths that I can use to feed positively into the problem going forward?

Hardworking—When I know what I need to do, I always do it.

Insight—At some level I know what I need to do here, I just need to be clearer.

Honesty—especially with self around weaknesses. Can be warm and accepting with clients, need to apply that to myself.

MY PROBLEM FORMULATION, INCLUDING VULNERABILITY FACTORS AND UNDERLYING PATTERNS

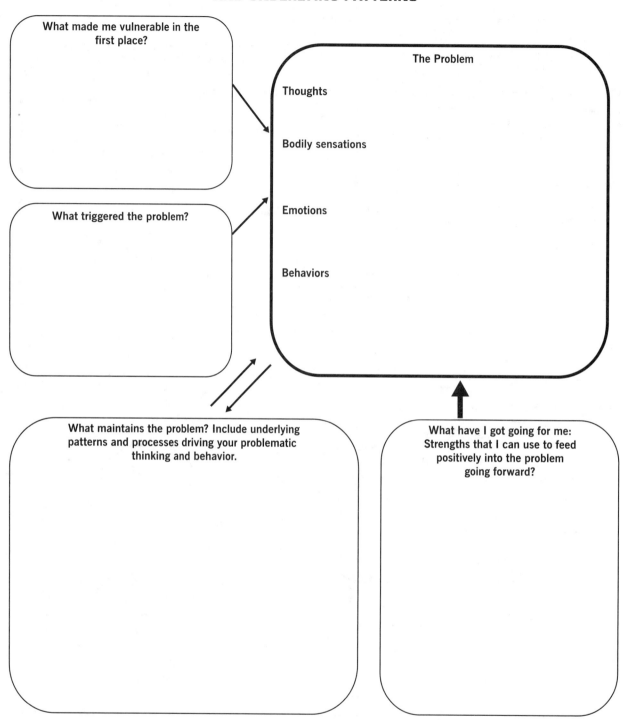

What made me vulnerable in the first place?

What triggered the problem?

The Problem

Thoughts

Bodily sensations

Emotions

Behaviors

What maintains the problem? Include underlying patterns and processes driving your problematic thinking and behavior.

What have I got going for me: Strengths that I can use to feed positively into the problem going forward?

Self-Reflective Questions

Comment on the process of testing out your thoughts using the thought record. Elaborate on any difficulties. Was the process helpful/unhelpful? Was the modified perspective convincing? At a head level—and also at a gut level (or not)?

_____

_____

_____

_____

_____

_____

_____

_____

_____

_____

_____

_____

_____

_____

_____

Have you noticed any changes in your thinking from doing the thought record exercise? What might you need to build into your personal or professional life to help you maintain your new way of thinking? (What situations might most challenge this?)

_____

_____

_____

_____

_____

_____

_____

_____

_____

_____

_____

_____

Comment on the use of Socratic questions to evaluate the problematic underlying patterns. How useful was this? Why, or why not? Was there any particular type of Socratic question that might be useful for you and your ways of thinking in the future?

_____

_____

_____

_____

_____

_____

_____

_____

_____

_____

_____

_____

_____

Going back to the client that you identified as giving you difficulty in the last module: if you are able to modify your own personal maintenance cycle, how will this affect your attitude or approach toward this particular client. What will you be doing differently in your sessions? What will this look and feel like?

_____

_____

_____

_____

_____

_____

_____

_____

_____

_____

_____

_____

What did you learn about yourself as a person and as a therapist from completing the expanded Problem Formulation diagram? Were there any surprises?

_____

_____

_____

_____

_____

_____

_____

_____

_____

_____

_____

_____

Did you notice any cultural or religious/spiritual influences? Can you describe these and comment on how influential they might have been.

_____

_____

_____

_____

_____

_____

_____

_____

_____

_____

_____

_____

_____

_____

Is there anything else you've noticed that you think it might be important to remember and come back to later?

_____

_____

_____

_____

_____

_____

_____

_____

_____

_____

_____

_____

MODULE 6

Reviewing Progress

I have learned such a lot from this module and feel so much more empathy for clients who really struggle to stick with treatment. It has highlighted the great importance of continuity and regular sessions—once the momentum is gone it's really hard to get it back. I have an experience now that I can share with clients when the going gets tough for them . . . and I will certainly be doing a more regular review of goals and goal measurements with clients.

—SP/SR participant

You are now about half-way through the SP/SR workbook. Completing the workbook is sometimes hard, as the process of paying attention to difficult thoughts and feelings can be demanding and tiring. We all have a range of demands competing for our time and even things that are important can get pushed down the priority list. We know that even with the best intentions people can drop out of SP/SR just as clients can struggle to stay with a course of therapy. This module aims to review where you are at with SP/SR so far and provides an opportunity to refocus if you've struggled to engage as much as you would have liked. In addition to considering factors around your engagement with the workbook, this module is also an opportune time to be considering the wider issues involved in practicing CBT on yourself.

Goal Review

First, it is important to remind yourself of the goals you set back at the start of the SP/SR workbook. This reminder will help you to refocus your attention and allow you to review your goals and identify any blocks to achieving them.

EXERCISE. Reviewing My Goals

Bring to mind the goal-setting imagery exercise you completed in Module 2 and your refined SMART goals. Complete the form on page 139.

REVIEWING MY GOALS

	Goal 1	Goal 2
Comment on your progress with each goal in general and in relation to the time frames you set for yourself. Are they as realistic and achievable as you originally thought? Are they measurable?		
Identify any roadblocks to achieving your goals: • Internal factors (e.g., your self-doubt, low motivation, old patterns of procrastination, self-criticism) • External factors over which you have some control (e.g., business, family demands) • External factors outside of your control		
Were you able to predict the roadblocks in Module 2? Were the strategies you developed adequate? What can you do to get around these roadblocks? Do you need to adjust your goals?		
Refine or rewrite your goals as necessary in light of this review.		

139

✍️ **EXERCISE.** Reviewing My Problem Using the Visual Analogue Scale

Refer back to the VAS that you used to rate the challenging problem in Module 1. Rate your level of distress now on the scale below.

0% —————————————— 50% —————————————— 100%

Not present   Moderate   Most severe

What has been the range of severity over the last 2 weeks [least intense to most intense distress]?

_____% to _____%

How does this compare to your ratings in Module 1? What do you make of this? Note your observations in the box below.

MY CHALLENGING PROBLEM: REFLECTIONS ON PROGRESS TO DATE

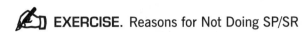 **EXERCISE.** Reasons for Not Doing SP/SR

The form below is an adaptation of the *Reasons for Not Doing Self-Help Assignments*, developed by Aaron T. Beck, John Rush, Brian Shaw, and Gary Emery for use with their clients. We have adapted the questions for SP/SR rather than for therapy. Read the statements and circle any that apply to you in relation to your completion of the SP/SR activities to date.

REASONS FOR NOT COMPLETING SP/SR ASSIGNMENTS

1. I'm happy with my skills as a therapist and there is no reason to change them.

2. I really can't see the point of doing SP/SR.

3. I feel that SP/SR will not be helpful. It really doesn't make good sound sense to me.

4. I think to myself, "I am a procrastinator, therefore I can't do this." And so I end up not doing it.

5. I am willing to do some self-help assignments, but I keep forgetting.

6. I do not have enough time, I am too busy.

7. If I do SP/SR as suggested here, it's not as good as if I come up with my own ideas.

8. I feel helpless, and I don't really believe that I can do things that I want to.

9. I have the feeling that the SP/SR program is trying to shape the way I think about therapy.

10. I don't feel like cooperating with the program.

11. I fear disapproval or criticism of my work. I believe that what I do just won't be good enough.

12. I have no desire or motivation to do SP/SR modules or anything else. Since I don't feel like doing these modules, it follows that I can't do them and I should not have to do them.

13. I feel too bad, sad, nervous, upset (pick appropriate words) to do it now.

14. I am feeling good now and I don't want to spoil it by working on the SP/SR program.

15. It feels too exposing.

16. Other reasons (please write them below).

_____

_____

_____

_____

EXERCISE. Identifying Roadblocks to Your Program

For both clients and therapists there may be issues or experiences that get in the way of making progress with therapy or training programs. In the box below, list anything that has interfered with your progress, including both internal factors (thoughts, emotions, time management, and so on) and external factors.

ROADBLOCKS TO PROGRESS

Have you identified any other roadblocks to progress—for example, automatic thoughts (about yourself or the workbook), negative beliefs about yourself, anxiety due to self-consciousness, procrastination, poor planning or time management, managing the demands of others on your time? Comment below.

Problem Solving

Working with our clients to help them learn how to identify and elucidate roadblocks or problems is often a CBT intervention in itself. Thereafter we can begin to identify, evaluate, and implement possible solutions when they feel stuck or unsure of what action to take.

Problem solving is one of the core CBT strategies. The purpose of the next exercise is to use any *barriers* that you have identified to fully engaging with SP/SR as an opportunity to practice problem-solving strategies.

✍ EXERCISE. My Problem Solving

First have a look at Jayashri's problem solving example below and on pages 144–145. Then use the problem-solving worksheet on pages 146–147 to address one of your barriers to participating in SP/SR.

> After reflecting on her Reasons for Not Completing SP/SR Assignments questionnaire, Jayashri identified that one of her beliefs was, "There is no point in doing SP/SR, I'll never be able to change." It was not that she did not recognize that she had a problem or that her goals were wrong, she had just started to feel helpless and to have thoughts that there was no point in trying to change this. In addition, she recognized that she had managed to "get by" so far with her current way of being and did not want to "rock the boat" by making big changes.
>
> She also identified that she was struggling to identify adequate time to engage with SP/SR: she was finding that, despite her good intentions each week, she found herself rushing through the tasks and then barely having time to reflect on the implications of her self-practice.
>
> In the form on pages 144–145, you can see how Jayashri has used this set of beliefs and behaviors as an input to problem solving.

JAYASHRI'S PROBLEM-SOLVING WORKSHEET

Step 1. Problem Identification: Define the problem in factual terms using simple language.

I have a belief that it's hopeless to try and change and that I'll never manage it.

Strangely I can recognize a contradictory belief that I've managed okay with my current beliefs, and that it would be risky to try and rock the boat now.

(Interesting that these two beliefs almost contradict each other: On the one hand, I don't think I can change and, on the other, I am scared that I might change! Both beliefs lead me to avoid doing the SP/SR work and I find myself leaving it to the last minute and not giving it the attention I need to in order to benefit from it.)

I haven't got enough time to spend on SP/SR in my current week, I am engaging less and feeling less hopeful about the benefits.

Problem summary

I am not spending very much time on SP/SR; this is reducing how much benefit I am getting from it and also limits my hope that I will be able to change my target problem.

Step 2. Brainstorm Solutions: Come up with as many options as possible. Don't reject/censor any options yet!

—Give up SP/SR.

—Set time aside on a weekend and stick rigidly to it.

—Swop the problem I am working on to pick something that I am less scared of or less ambivalent about.

—Speak to my colleague who is also doing SP/SR to see what she thinks and how she is managing.

—Discuss things with my supervisor.

—Ask my boss for study leave each week for SP/SR.

—Ensure I finish my clinical work and note-keeping on time one night per week and stay a little later so I can set aside some time for SP/SR.

Step 3. Strengths and Weaknesses Analysis: Choose two or three of the most promising possibilities and do a strengths and weaknesses analysis.

Solution	Strengths	Weaknesses
Give up SP/SR	I will immediately have a spare 2 hours per week to spend on other things. I won't feel guilty each week for not doing the work.	I will remain stuck with my current problem. I won't make any changes in my personal life. and I've already started to notice how much I need to. I will feel like a failure.
Ensure I finish work on time one night per week and stay a little later so I can allocate time for SP/SR.	This is something I have wanted to do for a long time and would be a good habit to get into. This would force me to reduce my note-keeping (which I have been told is over the top in length and detail). It won't reduce my free time out of work.	Finishing on time has been difficult for me to achieve in the past. I need a better plan here. Colleagues at work might pop in to have a chat and disturb my "flow" when working on my SP/SR.

Step 4. Solution Selection: Select a solution to try based on this analysis.

Okay, it makes sense to carve out time for SP/SR straight after work. I can achieve two aims in one, address my late working and free up time to work on SP/SR outside of my current free time.

Step 5. Implementation Planning: Outline your plan of action. What steps will you take to apply your solution?

I will ensure I don't book any clients in past 4 P.M.

I will have a look at some colleagues' notes and look for ideas on how I can cut mine down and save time.

I will tell my colleagues of my plans and that, while I may be at work during that time, I'm not to be disturbed unless it is really important.

I will take my SP/SR workbook to my office and clear a place in my locked cabinet.

When will you begin?

I can start to make some changes tomorrow but realistically it won't be until next week that I can implement all of the steps.

What problems might you encounter? How will you overcome these?
What resources do you need (e.g., help from someone else)?

I might be tired and will want to go home even if I manage to finish on time.

I will stay late at work and complete the workbook before going home even if I only spend 30 minutes on it. I might be tired but I will still be in a focused mode and will then reward myself by buying takeout on the way home!

I will tell my colleague and Anish what I am doing, which will make it harder for me to change my mind.

MY PROBLEM-SOLVING WORKSHEET

Step 1. Problem Identification: Define the problem in factual terms using simple language.

Problem summary

Step 2. Brainstorm Solutions: Come up with as many options as possible. Don't reject/censor any options yet!

Step 3. Strengths and Weaknesses Analysis: Choose two or three of the most promising possibilities and do a strengths and weaknesses analysis.

Solution	Strengths	Weaknesses

Step 4. Solution Selection: Select a solution to try based on this analysis.

Step 5. Implementation Planning: Outline your plan of action. What steps will you take to apply your solution?

When will you begin?

What problems might you encounter? How will you overcome these?
What resources do you need (e.g., help from someone else)?

It is helpful to review how your problem-solving strategy is working once you have tried it for a few days. After 5–7 days (or thereabouts), complete Steps 6 and 7 to check if you need to make any adjustments to your strategy.

MY PROBLEM-SOLVING WORKSHEET REVIEW

Step 6. Implementation: What did you do? Write exactly what you did.
Step 7. Review: How did it go? Write below how well your solution worked. If it is not working, or the results are not satisfactory, go back to Step 4 and pick another solution to try. And/ or review any negative beliefs you have about your problem-solving abilities, as these may be interfering in the process particularly if you are a "worrier."

Self-Reflective Questions

You have now completed half of the workbook. How would you summarize your overall reaction to the self-practice exercises thus far? Is there a difference between what you have experienced at a rational intellectual level and what you may have felt at a "gut level"?

_____

_____

_____

_____

_____

_____

_____

_____

_____

_____

_____

_____

_____

_____

_____

_____

Have any of your experiences of self-practice particularly stood out for you? If so, how would you account for this?

_____

_____

_____

_____

_____

_____

_____

_____

_____

_____

_____

_____

_____

This module has focused on reviewing your SP/SR progress and identifying roadblocks. Have you discovered anything about yourself in this context? Did you notice any self-criticism relating to your engagement with SP/SR? If so, how did this feel? Are there any ways that you could use this as an opportunity to relate to yourself in a different (e.g., more compassionate) way?

_____

_____

_____

_____

_____

_____

_____

_____

_____

_____

_____

_____

When you consider the impact of the SP/SR thus far, have you experienced this as mainly affecting your "personal self" or your "therapist self," or both? How do you think your personal and professional learnings relate to one another?

_____

_____

_____

_____

_____

_____

_____

_____

_____

_____

_____

Can you bring to mind a particular client who may be experiencing difficulty in progressing? Is there anything that you have learned from reviewing your own progress that might be relevant for this client? If so, how will you put this into practice? When? Where? How?

_____

_____

_____

_____

_____

_____

_____

_____

_____

_____

_____

_____

_____

_____

What has been your reaction to the self-reflective questions at the end of each module? Can you identify any difficulties with the reflective process? Are there any steps you can take to improve this experience for yourself?

_____

_____

_____

_____

_____

_____

_____

_____

_____

_____

_____

_____

_____

Is there anything else you've noticed in this module that you think might be important to remember and come back to later?

_____

_____

_____

_____

_____

_____

_____

_____

_____

_____

_____

PART II

Creating and Strengthening
New Ways of Being

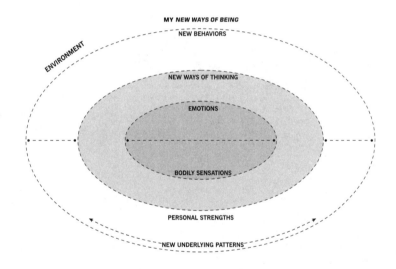

Identifying Unhelpful Assumptions and Constructing New Alternatives

*I've become a great deal more aware of patients using the if/
then prompts and I feel it has made me identify things much
easier than I did before. I've also identified it more in myself.*
                                                    —SP/SR participant

In Part I of the workbook, "Identifying and Understanding *Unhelpful (Old) Ways of Being*," the self-practice CBT interventions have been largely focused on your challenging problem. The aim was first to understand and find an explanation for how and why your problem kept reoccurring; then to develop a problem statement and identify measurable, realistic, and achievable goals. You went on to build the formulation further, and to find ways to modify the cognitive content and underlying patterns of thought and behavior. These exercises have hopefully empowered you to experiment with a variety of interventions to change unhelpful ways of being. It is also relevant that, alongside the challenging problem, you have already been considering your strengths. Your strengths will come into sharper focus in the SP exercises in the second half of the workbook.

In Part II of the workbook, "Creating and Strengthening *New Ways of Being*," we shall be adopting a complementary set of strategies that emphasize a strengths focus rather than a problem focus. These strategies tend to be more experiential: imagery and behavioral experiments are particularly prominent. Experiential strategies to build *New Ways of Being* have been gaining momentum in the past few years through the influence of cognitive science, clinical innovation within CBT, and positive psychology.

Up to this point in the workbook, you have been working with the most accessible level of thought, namely, automatic thoughts. As we work toward creating *New Ways of Being,* our focus shifts to a deeper, less accessible level of thought: underlying assumptions, attitudes, and "rules for living" that may impact on us across a variety of different situations (e.g., "If I perform extremely well at all times, people may not realize how flawed I really am"). The aim over the next six modules is to find further ways to undermine the old unhelpful patterns of thinking, feeling, and behaving; and to build new strengths-based *Ways of Being*, which can empower you in both your personal and professional life.

We highlight four interrelated strategies to create *New Ways of Being*:

1. Identifying unhelpful *Old Ways of Being*, especially old behavioral patterns and underlying assumptions (e.g., "If I am really nice to all my clients, they may not see what an incompetent therapist I am"). This is an important first step because it is important to understand why our old unhelpful ways of thinking, feeling, and behaving continue.
2. Constructing potential *New Ways of Being* by asking, "How would I like to be?"
3. Contrasting *Unhelpful (Old) Ways of Being* with *New Ways of Being*.
4. Strengthening *New Ways of Being*, particularly through the use of experiential strategies such as behavioral experiments and imagery-based techniques.

The current module is predominantly focused on (1) self-practice exercises to identify your underlying assumptions and behavioral patterns associated with your *Old Ways of Being* and (2) techniques to construct more helpful assumptions or rules to live by, and to develop more adaptive patterns of thinking and behavior.

Modules 8 and 9 contrast *Old* and *New Ways of Being*, and start to strengthen *New Ways of Being*. Strategies to strengthen the *New Ways of Being* are the focus of Modules 10 and 11. The final module, Module 12, aims to consolidate your *New Ways of Being* so that you are in a position to continue their development beyond the end of the program.

Underlying Assumptions

Briefly summarized, classical cognitive-behavioral theory identifies three different, but related levels of thought: automatic thoughts, underlying assumptions, and core beliefs. Core beliefs are unconditional, absolutist beliefs about ourselves, other people, and the world. Core beliefs are usually not consciously accessible but may influence our behavior and emotional reactions across a wide range of situations (e.g., "I am unlovable," "Other people are untrustworthy," "The world is unpredictable").

Classical cognitive-behavioral theory views underlying assumptions as an intermediate layer of thought between core beliefs and automatic thoughts. The theory suggests that underlying assumptions "help us to cope" with the implications of our core beliefs ("I'm worthless, so I *must* _____ so people do not notice how [. . .] I am"). Underlying assumptions can often be phrased as "*if . . . , then. . . .*" statements, or "musts," "shoulds," or "oughts." Typically they impact upon our emotions, thoughts, and behavior across different situations.

Underlying assumptions can be positive or negative, helpful or unhelpful. They are frequently unquestioned rules for living that have been learned from family, friends, workplaces, or school (e.g. "If people are nasty to you, be nasty back!"). Although classical cognitive behavioral theory has tied underlying assumptions closely to core beliefs, there is a growing recognition that our rules for living or operating principles are not necessarily tied to core beliefs. For instance, as therapists we develop some quite specific "rules for therapy," unrelated to our core beliefs (e.g., "If a client expresses clear suicidal plans, I must let the following people know. . .", and may have some beliefs that are quite situation-specific and often realistic (e.g., "I'm doing okay with clients with anxiety problems, but struggling with my clients who are severely depressed").

Summary: The Three Levels of Thought

Automatic Thoughts

- Are situation-specific.
- Pop into our minds.
- Coexist with our more deliberate thinking.
- Typically tend to be slightly out of awareness.
- Connect to emotion.
- Can be biased by distorted interpretations and are seldom evaluated.

Underlying Assumptions

- Are cross-situational assumptions, operating principles, or rules for living about self, others, or the world.
- May or may not be derived from core beliefs.
- Can be expressed as "if . . . , then . . ." conditional statements, or "musts," "shoulds," or "oughts."
- Connect beliefs with behaviors and emotions.

Core Beliefs

- Are strongly held cross-situational unconditional absolute beliefs about self, others, and the world.
- Can be helpful or unhelpful.
- Their development is often influenced by childhood experience with influential significant others and/or by trauma experiences.

In *Experiencing CBT from the Inside Out* our focus is on automatic thoughts and underlying assumptions, rather than core beliefs. On the theoretical and practical grounds that we have articulated in Chapters 2 and 3, we neither regard it as necessary nor desirable for therapists using this workbook to be working at the core belief level. *Experiencing CBT from the Inside Out* has not been designed for in-depth psychotherapy!

Underlying assumptions can be quite subtle and difficult to detect but we can find clues in our characteristic compensatory behaviors, and underlying patterns of thought and emotion such as emotional avoidance and safety behaviors. You will already be familiar with some of your unhelpful compensatory behavioral responses from completing Module 4 and may be able to deduce some of your therapist-related assumptions from these.

 EXAMPLE: Shelly's and David's Underlying Assumptions

In the early stages of her training, Shelly had a therapist belief, "I am no good as a therapist." To cope with this belief, the underlying assumption guiding her behavior was: "If I avoid observation of my therapy sessions, then my supervisor will not know what a poor therapist I am." Consequently, Shelly avoided observation of her sessions by her supervisor. She did this by making excuses and missing supervision appointments.

David was feeling insecure regarding his knowledge of CBT. So he began to wonder if he was "a good-enough therapist" (belief about self as therapist), thinking "my young supervisor is judging me negatively" (belief about others). This led to the assumption, "If I show her how experienced and knowledgeable I am, then she will recognize my experience and skill." Behaviorally David acted in accordance with his underlying assumption by continually making reference to other models of therapy that he had used successfully in the past and indulging in long justifications about how and why he may have made certain clinical decisions. His behavior had the contradictory effect of irritating rather than impressing his supervisor.

The Gateway to Identifying Our Unhelpful Underlying Assumptions: Recurring Personal Themes, Compensatory Behaviors, and Avoidance Behaviors

As we have already seen, underlying assumptions can be elusive. As CBT therapists, we play an important role in helping our clients to identify their assumptions or rules for living. A gateway to their assumptions is provided through several key strategies: recurring personal themes, compensatory behaviors, and avoidance behaviors. To open the gate for ourselves in the context of this workbook we can:

1. Search for *recurring personal themes* (e.g., themes of being rejected, challenging authority, or being put to the test). Themes can be found in our habitual cognitive, behavioral, and emotional responses.
2. Gain awareness of our *compensatory behaviors*, which typically take the form of *repetitive behaviors and rigid coping strategies*: the kind of behaviors we feel we *always* have to do.
3. Gain awareness of our *avoidance behaviors*.

The next set of self-practice exercises focuses on these three areas. Recurring personal themes, compensatory behaviors, and avoidance behaviors provide the clues from which we can deduce the rules that guide important aspects of our lives.

Identifying Recurring Personal Themes

This exercise, focused on personal themes, will help to pull together your learning from the first six modules.

 EXAMPLE: Shelly's Recurring Personal Themes

Using the simple form on page 162, Shelly set about identifying some of the emotions, thoughts, bodily sensations, and behaviors that were recurring features of her supervision sessions.

ONE OF SHELLY'S RECURRING PERSONAL THEMES

Triggering situation(s)	Thoughts	Emotions/ bodily sensations	Behaviors including avoiding (people, places, emotions, circumstances)
An upcoming supervision session	I will be judged as not being up to scratch. I forgot to assess risk. My client might harm herself and it will be my fault.	Anxious Tense Self-doubt Guilt	Making an excuse that I could not get the camera to record. Ruminating about what I failed to do in the session.

 EXERCISE. My Recurring Personal Themes

Refer back to the exercises that you have completed so far, for example, your five-part formulation (Module 2) and the exercises to identify your unhelpful patterns of thought and behavior (Module 4). What are some of the repetitive triggers, cognitions, emotions, and behaviors that you have identified in relation to your challenging problem? Use the recurring themes form on page 162 to list them.

Note: If you feel you have satisfactorily resolved the problem you identified in Part I of the workbook and would like to focus on a new problem, please do so. You will need to understand the components of this new problem area by applying the five-part formulation from Module 2 and engaging with some of the other strategies (e.g., from Modules 4 and 5) before proceeding to the next tasks.

MY RECURRING PERSONAL THEMES

Triggering situation(s)	Thoughts	Emotions/bodily sensations	Behaviors including avoiding (people, places, emotions, circumstances)

Identifying Compensatory Behaviors:
Repetitive Behaviors and Rigid Coping Strategies

The focus of this exercise is on behaviors and coping strategies that are repetitive and compensatory in the sense that these behaviors "compensate" for unwanted feelings or thoughts. Recurrent behaviors and rigid coping strategies are classic compensatory behaviors. You have already identified some of these in Module 4. At this stage, leave aside avoidance behaviors, which will be addressed in the next section. In the box below are some examples of repetitive behaviors and rigid coping strategies. You may recognize some of these patterns as your own.

Examples of Repetitive Behaviors and Rigid Coping Strategies

- Trying to do everything perfectly.
- Seeking reassurance from others.
- Blaming other people when things go wrong.
- Finding it difficult to end therapy sessions on time.
- Trying to please others.
- Getting upset if a client terminates therapy unexpectedly or cancels appointments.
- Finding it hard to say no to others.
- Eating or drinking too much.
- Getting quite upset when I get any feedback that I think is negative.
- Hiding my true feelings.
- Finding it difficult to stand up for myself.
- Having a hard time making decisions.
- Working very long hours.

 EXERCISE. My Repetitive Behaviors and Rigid Coping Strategies

---

MY REPETITIVE BEHAVIORS AND RIGID COPING STRATEGIES

What are examples of my repetitive behaviors or rigid coping strategies?

Repetitive behaviors can give us clues to the form of our underlying assumptions. We engage with them because we think they will help us. Identifying them can help us to formulate the "if" part of an underlying assumption ("If I. . . .").

 EXAMPLE: David's Underlying Assumptions

> *If I let my supervisor know how experienced I am by telling her about the therapy models I have used* [behavior], *then she will respect me* [consequence].
>
> *If I explain in detail why I took a certain action* [behavior], *then she will take me seriously* [consequence].
>
> *If my supervisor asks me to explain a therapeutic decision* [behavior], *then she is questioning my CBT knowledge* [consequence].

EXERCISE. My Underlying Assumptions

If (behavior) _____

_____ ,

then _____

_____ (consequence).

If (behavior) _____

_____ ,

then _____

_____ (consequence).

If (behavior) _____

_____ ,

then _____

_____ (consequence).

Identifying Avoidance Behaviors

Avoidance is a behavior, even when that avoidance is of something internal (e.g., our emotions). We avoid situations, people, thoughts, emotions, and bodily sensations in an attempt to protect ourselves from experiencing pain or difficulties. For example, if I believe I am not good at working with specific types of client, I might avoid taking those referrals.

The box below lists some examples of avoidant behavior.

Examples of Avoidance Behaviors

- Trying not to think about upsetting things.
- Playing computer games or surfing the Internet for long periods.
- Withdrawing when there is interpersonal conflict.
- Withdrawing from people when I feel hurt.
- Watching a lot of TV.
- Going shopping.
- Eating when upset.
- Using alcohol or drugs.
- Daydreaming.

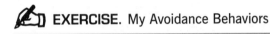 **EXERCISE.** My Avoidance Behaviors

MY AVOIDANCE BEHAVIORS

Identify any avoidance behaviors that you can recognize in yourself.

These patterns of avoidance behaviors, like repetitive behaviors, may form the "*if*" clause of an unhelpful underlying assumption. See if they help to identify any assumption(s) below.

If I (do that which I am avoiding) _____

_____,

then _____

_____.

If I (do that which I am avoiding) _____

_____,

then _____

_____.

If I (do that which I am avoiding) _____

_____,

then _____

_____.

EXERCISE. My Underlying Assumptions and Compensatory
and Avoidance Behaviors

Look back over this module and reflect on the self-practice exercises you have completed so far. On page 167, list the underlying assumptions that you have identified, the compensatory behaviors (e.g., repetitive behaviors, rigid coping strategies), and the avoidance behaviors.

Underlying assumptions	Associated compensatory (repetitive behaviors, rigid coping strategies) and/or avoidance behaviors

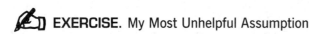 **EXERCISE.** My Most Unhelpful Assumption

Looking at these assumptions, consider which has the greatest negative influence on you in either a personal or a professional capacity. In Module 8, you will have the opportunity to test out this assumption against a more helpful new alternative.

For example, Shelly considered her most unhelpful old assumption to be: "If I avoid my supervisor's observation, then he will never know what a useless therapist I am."

MY MOST UNHELPFUL ASSUMPTION

What is your most unhelpful assumption? Add this below.

If _____

_____,

then _____

_____.

Creating New Alternative Assumptions

The final set of tasks in this module focuses on creating a set of new alternative assumptions and new patterns of thought and behavior that can provide the foundation for your *New Ways of Being*. As we shall see in the following modules, one of the key questions is: "How would I like . . . to feel? . . . to be thinking about myself? . . . to be doing things differently?

 EXAMPLE: Shelly's New Alternative Assumption

Shelly considered how she would like to be thinking about herself on a day-to-day basis in order to feel better about herself and her work. This required a quiet space for her to ponder how she would like to feel and a leap of imagination, but after a little time, she identified a new underlying assumption: "Although I'm not a perfect therapist, I know that I'm good enough. If I let my supervisor see what I do, he'll give me feedback and I know I can use this to improve."

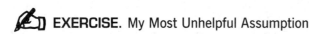 **EXERCISE.** Creating a New Alternative Assumption

How would I like to feel? How would I like to be thinking about myself, others, and the world? How would I like to be doing things? See if you can come up with one or more alternative underlying assumptions or rules that indicate how you would like to be. Add them in the box on page 169.

MY NEW ALTERNATIVE ASSUMPTION

Creating New Patterns of Thought and Behavior

Have a look at the compensatory and avoidance behaviors that you have identified and consider what kinds of helpful underlying patterns of thought and behavior might underpin your new assumptions or rules.

 EXAMPLE: Shelly's New Patterns of Thought and Behavior

Shelly projected herself into the future, and imagined what she would need to do to embed her new underlying assumption into *New Ways of Being*, and establish a positive maintenance cycle. She saw herself as:

- Adopting an approach orientation (not avoidance) toward supervisors, colleagues, and clients in order to test out what would really happen rather than just guessing.
- Experiencing her negative thoughts as just "phenomena" or "habit," not necessarily to be believed or acted upon.
- Specifically focusing her attention on things she is doing well.
- Being compassionate and gentle with herself when she doesn't get things right. The inevitable mistakes would then be less aversive and more of a learning experience.

 EXERCISE. Creating My New Patterns

Project yourself into the future and imagine what you will need to be doing, feeling, and thinking if your new underlying assumption is to become a reality. What kinds of new patterns of thinking and behavior will take the place of the old patterns? What kinds of images or thoughts about yourself or others will be helpful? Allow your imagination to roam. If it is too hard to imagine yourself in this context, you could try imagining that it is someone else (e.g., a close friend or colleague) in order to gain access to the kinds of cognition and behaviors that are likely to support your new underlying assumption.

MY NEW PATTERNS OF THOUGHT AND BEHAVIOR

Add your ideas below:

💭 *Self-Reflective Questions*

How did you experience the process of identifying your underlying assumptions? Did you have any particular emotional, behavioral, bodily, or cognitive responses? Did you experience any difficulty? Were there any surprises?

_____

_____

_____

_____

_____

_____

_____

_____

_____

_____

_____

_____

_____

Did you observe any personal themes that help you understand yourself more as a person and/or as a therapist? Have these exercises made any difference to your awareness of these themes?

_____

_____

_____

_____

_____

_____

_____

_____

_____

_____

_____

_____

_____

Are there any particular clients or people who routinely trigger your unhelpful assumptions? Can you understand why this may be happening? Is there anything you would like to do differently if this is the case? (It might be helpful to map this difficulty out as a maintenance cycle.)

_____

_____

_____

_____

_____

_____

_____

_____

_____

_____

_____

_____

Can you see any connections between your "therapist assumptions" and your "personal assumptions"? How do you understand these connections? What are the implications?

_____

_____

_____

_____

_____

_____

_____

_____

_____

_____

_____

_____

What was it like identifying an alternative, or *new*, more helpful assumption? How much did you believe the *new* assumption with your "head"? Did your "gut"—or "heart"—take a different view? If there was a difference, what sense do you make of this?

_____

_____

_____

_____

_____

_____

_____

_____

_____

_____

_____

_____

_____

How might your experience affect the way in which you help clients identify their underlying assumptions?

_____

_____

_____

_____

_____

_____

_____

_____

_____

_____

_____

What are the key things that you would like to remember from this module? Make a list of any points that you would like to recall when you see your next clients.

_____

_____

_____

_____

_____

_____

_____

_____

Using Behavioral Experiments to Test Unhelpful Assumptions against New Alternatives

> I have learned easier ways of recognizing when a behavioral experiment could be helpful and that it can be simple. Also that it doesn't have to be a one off. Patients can be afraid of anything and anything can be tested!! Right?! One of the biggest things that has come up from this is emphasis on rating and rerating. I tend to avoid this because it is fussy. Little did I know how it helps shift thoughts.
>
> —SP/SR participant

Behavioral experiments provide a chance for clients to learn directly from their *own* experience by testing out their assumptions and beliefs in day-to-day situations between sessions, or sometimes during sessions. While behavioral experiments are often anxiety-provoking, clinical experience and research suggests that they are one of the most powerful methods of change in CBT and can lead to significant therapeutic benefit.

Behavioral experiments are usually designed with one of three main purposes in mind:

1. To elaborate on the formulation (does the experiment add new information?)
2. To test negative beliefs about self, others, or the world (how accurate is my "old" perspective?)
3. To test new more adaptive beliefs (is there any evidence to support a new, more adaptive perspective?)

Behavioral experiments are particularly useful for testing out rules for living and assumptions to see whether they hold up in reality.

It is helpful to think about behavioral experiments as "no lose" endeavors. The nature of any experiment is that the outcome is unknown, so it is important to remain open to all possibilities. In approaching a behavioral experiment, the attitude we want to engender is that it will be valuable whatever the outcome; even an apparently disappointing outcome can lead to new information or more detailed information that can inform effective problem solving. This is what is meant by a "no lose" approach.

As a step toward formulating and contrasting your *Old Ways of Being* and the *New Ways of Being* in Module 9, in this module you will be planning and carrying out a behavioral experiment. The experiment will be designed to test an "old" unhelpful assumption (see purpose 2 above), and will also give you a chance to compare the old assumption with a potentially more helpful new assumption (see purpose 3 above). This module is also a precursor to Module 11, where you will be designing a behavioral experiment specifically to build evidence for your *New Ways of Being*.

During this module we ask you to rate your strength of belief in two ways: at a "gut" level and at a rational or "head" level. There is a good theoretical and practical rationale for making this distinction. Clients often say things like: "Rationally I know there is nothing to be afraid of, but at a gut level I'm terrified!" There is some evidence that certain types of interventions are more effective than others in changing beliefs at a "gut" level; by being explicit about potential discrepancies, we can better understand the process of belief change and more helpfully target our interventions.

Planning the Behavioral Experiment

• Step 1: In this module you will be using the first three columns of the behavioral experiment record sheet (see pages 179–180) to help design a behavioral experiment to test one of your *Old Ways* underlying assumptions.

• Step 2: Once you have planned the experiment and identified how you will address any problems or barriers that might occur, it is time to carry it out.

• Step 3: At this stage you will review the experiment using the last two columns of the behavioral experiment record sheet to identify what occurred, what can be learned from it, and what future steps can be taken to consolidate any learning. This step is crucial in ensuring that maximum learning occurs from the experiment.

EXERCISE. My Behavioral Experiment Record Sheet

First, review Shelly's example on pages 177–178. Next, complete your own behavioral experiment record sheet on pages 179–180, comparing an *Old Ways* assumption with a *New Ways* assumption and troubleshooting potential problems in carrying it out.

> Shelly designed an experiment to test out her unhelpful assumption, "If I allow my supervisor to observe my therapy, then he will realize what a useless therapist I am" that was causing her a problem at work.
>
> For comparison purposes, she also developed a *New Ways* assumption: "Although I'm not a perfect therapist, I know that I'm good enough. If I let my supervisor see what I do, he'll think it's fine and will help me to improve."
>
> Although her belief in her *New Ways* assumption was very low, she recognized that it might be important to start the process of viewing her experience through a different lens.

SHELLY'S BEHAVIORAL EXPERIMENT RECORD SHEET (FIRST THREE COLUMNS)

Target cognition(s)	Experiment	Prediction(s)	Outcome	What I learned
What *Old Ways* thought, assumption or belief are you testing? Is there a *New Ways* assumption that you would prefer to believe and act on? Rate belief in cognitions (0–100%) first as a "gut-level" belief rating, then with "rational-mind" rating in parentheses.	Design an experiment to test out the *New Ways* idea (e.g., facing a situation you would otherwise avoid, dropping precautions, behaving in a new way). Where? When? With whom? What will you be looking out for?	What do you predict will happen? Make two sets of predictions, one based on your *Old Ways* assumptions, the other on your *New Ways* assumptions. How likely are these outcomes? Make "gut-level" and "rational-mind" ratings. (0–100%)	What actually happened? What did you observe about yourself (behavior, thoughts, feelings, bodily sensations)? About your environment, about other people? Any difficulties? What did you do about them? How does the outcome fit with your predictions?	How much do you now believe your original (*Old Ways*) and alternative (*New Ways*) assumptions (0–100%)? What have you learned about any safety behaviors? Will you be dropping them? What are the practical implications? Does your *New Ways* assumption need to be modified? If so, what might the modified version be?
Old Ways Assumption If I allow my supervisor to observe my therapy then he will realize what a useless therapist I am. 85% (40%)	During the next week I will take a recording of a therapy session to supervision. I will ask my supervisor to listen to a section that I need help with.	**Old Ways Prediction** I have an image of my supervisor sitting there looking stony faced, a look that tells me just how disappointed he is in me. I will be able to tell that he thinks I'm a useless therapist. 80% (30%)		**Belief Ratings:** **Old Ways Assumption** ____% (____%) **New Ways Assumption** ____% (____%)
New Ways Assumption Although I'm not a perfect therapist, I know that I'm good enough. If I let my supervisor see what I do, he'll think it's fine and will help me to improve. 10% (40%)		**New Ways Prediction** I know that I have effectively used feedback in the past. It's one of my strengths. I won't assume what he is thinking and will ask if I am not clear. I know I'm okay as a therapist and can cope with any negative feedback however uncomfortable. 30% (50%)		

Troubleshooting potential problems

What habitual (*Old Ways*) compensatory or safety behavior/s would you normally utilize to prevent what you think will be the worst outcome?

I might try and avoid recording a session and even if I do I might select the best bit and then pretend it's a bit where I'm struggling!

How will you prevent yourself from doing this?

I need to remind myself that I won't learn anything new if I don't do something new. I will make a specific plan.

What will you do instead?

Just notice the thoughts telling me to avoid, they are just thoughts, and it was these thoughts that have got me stuck in the first place. Ignore the old thoughts, do something new! I will take a chance and show him my therapy as it is. I will be honest with him and myself.

What problems may get in the way?

I might be tempted not to ask clients if I can record our sessions. Or I might have technical problems with my camera.

How will you deal with them?

I will commit to doing this during the week and if I have technical problems then I will arrange for my supervisor to sit in on a session.

MY BEHAVIORAL EXPERIMENT RECORD SHEET

Target cognition(s)	Experiment	Prediction(s)	Outcome	What I learned
What *Old Ways* thought, assumption or belief are you testing? Is there a *New Ways* assumption that you would prefer to believe and act on? Rate belief in cognitions (0–100%) first as a "gut-level" belief rating, then with "rational-mind" rating in parentheses.	Design an experiment to test out the *New Ways* idea (e.g., facing a situation you would otherwise avoid, dropping precautions, behaving in a new way). Where? When? With whom? What will you be looking out for?	What do you predict will happen? Make two sets of predictions, one based on your *Old Ways* assumptions, the other on your *New Ways* assumptions. How likely are these outcomes? Make "gut-level" and "rational-mind" ratings. (0–100%)	What actually happened? What did you observe about yourself (behavior, thoughts, feelings, bodily sensations)? About your environment, about other people? Any difficulties? What did you do about them? How does the outcome fit with your predictions?	How much do you now believe your original (*Old Ways*) and alternative (*New Ways*) assumptions (0–100%)? What have you learned about any safety behaviors? Will you be dropping them? What are the practical implications? Does your *New Ways* assumption need to be modified? If so, what might the modified version be?
Old Ways Assumption		*Old Ways Prediction*		**Belief Ratings:** *Old Ways Assumption* ___ % (___ %) *New Ways Assumption* ___ % (___ %)
New Ways Assumption		*New Ways Prediction*		

179

Troubleshooting potential problems

What habitual (*Old Ways*) compensatory or safety behavior/s would you normally utilize to prevent what you think will be the worst outcome?

How will you prevent yourself from doing this?

What will you do instead?

What problems may get in the way?

How will you deal with them?

Outcome of the Behavioral Experiment

After you have completed your behavioral experiment, take some time to think about what happened (and what did not happen) so you can complete the last two columns of the worksheet on page 179. These questions and headings will help you review the experience and pull together the information from the experiment into a format that you can use as you continue working on the relevant issue.

 EXERCISE. My Behavioral Experiment Review

> First, look at page 182 and see how Shelly's experiment went and how she made sense of what she observed. Note that she completed the fourth and fifth columns, "Outcome" and "What I learned." To make the most of her learning, she answered the key questions and rerated her belief in her assumptions.

Now note the outcome of your own experiment and what you learned in the fourth and fifth columns on page 179.

🍎 SHELLY'S BEHAVIORAL EXPERIMENT RECORD SHEET REVIEW

Target cognition(s)	Experiment	Prediction(s)	Outcome	What I learned
What *Old Ways* thought, assumption or belief are you testing? Is there a *New Ways* assumption that you would prefer to believe and act on? Rate belief in cognitions (0–100%) first as a "gut-level" belief rating, then with "rational-mind" rating in parentheses.	Design an experiment to test out the *New Ways* idea (e.g., facing a situation you would otherwise avoid, dropping precautions, behaving in a new way). Where? When? With whom? What will you be looking out for?	What do you predict will happen? Make two sets of predictions, one based on your *Old Ways* assumptions, the other on your *New Ways* assumptions. How likely are these outcomes? Make "gut-level" and "rational-mind" ratings. (0–100%)	What actually happened? What did you observe about yourself (behavior, thoughts, feelings, bodily sensations)? About your environment, about other people? Any difficulties? What did you do about them? How does the outcome fit with your predictions?	How much do you now believe your original (*Old Ways*) and alternative (*New Ways*) assumptions (0–100%)? What have you learned about any safety behaviors? Will you be dropping them? What are the practical implications? Does your *New Ways* assumption need to be modified? If so, what might the modified version be?
Old Ways Assumption If I allow my supervisor to observe my therapy then he will realize what a useless therapist I am. 85% (40%)	*During the next week I will take a recording of a therapy session to supervision. I will ask my supervisor to listen to a section that I need help with.*	**Old Ways Prediction** *I have an image of my supervisor sitting there looking stony faced, a look that tells me just how disappointed he is in me. I will be able to tell that he thinks I'm a useless therapist.* 80% (30%)	*I forced myself to record a session and I showed a random section to my supervisor. Admittedly I'd put off recording all week and only asked a client at the end of the week.* *I was very anxious about recording the session and felt a bit stiff and unnatural to start with and then soon forgot. When I arrived at supervision I felt anxious again and part of me wanted to avoid playing the recording. I had to stay strong in order to try and lead my supervisor into talking about a theoretical issue. As I started the tape I felt a little sick and really quite vulnerable. It reminded me of how much I hated sitting exams at school and how I always thought I was going to be "found out." It also got me thinking about how much of my time I worry about what other people think—both at work and outside of work . . . .*	**Belief Ratings:** **Old Ways Assumption** 35 % (30 %) **New Ways Assumption** 50 % (60 %) *I need to keep doing this. My unhelpful belief has been weakened but it isn't going to just disappear. It's okay to be "good enough." It's hard for me to write this but actually part of me does feel I'm quite a good therapist at times! My avoidance is actually stopping me from benefitting from supervision and making it harder to actually learn. It keeps me feeling like a poor therapist because I couldn't really get any specific feedback from my supervisor.* *How about each month I schedule situations where I fear being exposed and have a chance to get new information? I will definitely ask or answer a question at each training session I go to. As soon as I notice those old thoughts that I'm not good enough, I need to take a moment to calm myself and think: "what do I need to do this time rather than just going along with the thoughts?"*
New Ways Assumption Although I'm not a perfect therapist, I know that I'm good enough. If I let my supervisor see what I do, he'll think it's fine and will help me to improve. 10% (40%)		**New Ways Prediction** *I know that I have effectively used feedback in the past. It's one of my strengths. I won't assume what he is thinking and will ask if I am not clear. I know I'm okay as a therapist and can cope with any negative feedback however uncomfortable.* 30% (50%)		

Creating Follow-Up Experiments

Usually several experiments are needed to embed *New Ways of Being.* So it may be important to devise follow-up experiments. After completing her first experiment, Shelly realized that she needed to stop avoiding situations where she feared she would be judged. In the box below, Shelly devised plans for some follow-up experiments.

SHELLY'S FOLLOW-UP EXPERIMENTS: WHAT, WHERE, WITH WHOM?

First I will take a therapy recording to my group supervision; this is a major test for me! I also need to think about how I do things differently outside work as I think it's part of the same problem. I stay within my comfort zone all the time, trying to make sure I don't do anything that I'm not comfortable with—just to avoid people judging me. I even do this with people I'm close to. I realized that I don't even try and cook new recipes for Stevie in case they go wrong and she thinks I'm a terrible cook! I need to spend some time thinking about the different situations I need to experiment in, maybe I will start with situations with people I feel more confident with and then work up to things that seem harder (e.g., maybe starting a new exercise class rather than staying in my old one that I'm familiar with). I've always wanted to restart playing the piano that I gave up at school. I will plan to look into this in the next week.

Now it is your turn to devise some follow-up experiments

MY FOLLOW-UP EXPERIMENTS

Self-Reflective Questions

What did you notice about your experience as you were planning a behavioral experiment? (Emotions? Thoughts? Behaviors? Bodily reactions?)

_____

_____

_____

_____

_____

_____

_____

_____

_____

_____

_____

Were you fearful of the possibility of the *Old Ways* predictions coming true? Was there a difference in how much you believed in the likelihood of this outcome in your "head" or "rational mind" compared with your "heart" or "gut"?

_____

_____

_____

_____

_____

_____

_____

_____

_____

_____

_____

_____

What did you notice about your experience of actually carrying out the behavioral experiment? Was there anything that surprised you?

_____

_____

_____

_____

_____

_____

_____

_____

_____

_____

_____

_____

_____

What did you notice when you reflected on your behavioral experiment after the event and tried to make sense of what actually happened? Did you notice any "head–gut differences"?

_____

_____

_____

_____

_____

_____

_____

_____

_____

_____

_____

_____

What did you learn about yourself:

As a therapist?

_____

_____

_____

_____

_____

_____

_____

_____

_____

_____

_____

_____

As a person beyond your work situation?

_____

_____

_____

_____

_____

_____

_____

_____

_____

_____

_____

_____

How are you going to consolidate this learning? What might you need to do?

_____

_____

_____

_____

_____

_____

_____

_____

_____

_____

_____

_____

Try to bring to mind a specific client that has made an intellectual shift in his or her beliefs but is struggling to change his or her beliefs at a heart or gut level. How might you use a behavioral experiment to help this client to make that "gut-level" shift in belief?

_____

_____

_____

_____

_____

_____

_____

_____

_____

_____

_____

_____

_____

What strategies would you use to help your clients to learn most effectively from their experiments? Will this affect how you review behavioral experiments with them?

_____

_____

_____

_____

_____

_____

_____

_____

_____

_____

_____

_____

_____

_____

Constructing *New Ways of Being*

LOVED the *New Ways of Being* Record Book. . . . I was surprised at just how much stuff I had a tendency to ignore. Funny how I use these things with patients, and KNOW how useful they are, but never use them myself, because 'I don't need to.' I thought this was a fantastic way to end the module, to bring it full circle and highlight the negative bias still steering me back to my old way of being. And then smashing it to pieces!! Reflecting back on the old and new ways of being, I can see that I am now sitting more comfortably in the new.

—SP/SR participant

The next three modules feature a new concept, the *Ways of Being* model, which we have developed in the context of this workbook. The focus of Part I of the workbook was to identify and understand the *Old Ways of Being*. The focus of Part II is to develop and strengthen the *New Ways of Being*. *New Ways of Being* strategies emphasize a strengths focus rather than a problem focus; they also have a strongly experiential flavor. As we have described in greater detail in Chapter 2, the concept of *Old* and *New Ways of Being* has been derived from two principle sources: cognitive science and recent clinical innovations.

The cognitive science influences have been multilevel information-processing models, in particular John Teasdale and Philip Barnard's Interacting Cognitive Subsystems (ICS), which suggest that, at more automatic "deeper" levels of processing (e.g., underlying patterns, assumptions, rules for living, core beliefs), our thoughts, images, behavior, emotions, and bodily feelings are relatively undifferentiated, and tend to be experienced together as a "package": "wheeled in" and "wheeled out" in Teasdale and

Barnard's terms. The ICS model also points the way to the growing recognition among CBT therapists that experiential strategies, such as behavioral experiments and imagery, are central to creating "heart"- or "gut"-level change.

To reflect this more holistic understanding of the deeper levels of information processing, we have created for this workbook new formulation diagrams, which we call "disks." These *Old Ways of Being* and *New Ways of Being* "disks" consist of three concentric circles representing emotions/bodily sensations (within the same circle), cognitions, behaviors, and underlying patterns.

A second influence has been the clinical innovations of creative therapists such as Christine Padesky and Kathleen Mooney, Kees Korrelboom and colleagues, and Paul Gilbert; and the role of positive psychology in orienting therapy toward positive emotional states (not just the eradication of negative states). See Chapter 2, where these clinical innovations and their relationship to cognitive science are discussed in more detail.

✏️ EXERCISE. My *Old Ways of Being*

We start by formulating your *Old Ways of Being*. First, have a look at the example of Shelly's *Old Ways of Being* disk on page 192, and how she got there below.

> Shelly identified her emotions/bodily sensations, cognitions, behaviors, and unhelpful maintaining patterns. This took her a bit of time. She had to "go inside" to identify the emotions and bodily feelings, and she recalled the underlying patterns such as avoidance and safety behaviors, worry and rumination, and selective attention that had been keeping her stuck.
>
> Once she had noted her old ways of thinking (cognitions) in the middle circle of the disk, she rated her percentage belief in them (she used her prebehavioral experiment ratings to characterize her *Old Ways of Being*, since the behavioral experiment in Module 8 had already had some impact on her beliefs).

Now complete your *Old Ways of Being* disk on page 193. Do this before proceeding further with the instructions. Focus on the problems that you have identified, but if they have resolved, you might like to extend these to any other work- or personal-related problems that you have noticed in the meantime. Think about specific situations to help generate your cognitions that might be in the form of automatic thoughts, underlying assumptions, or therapist and/or personal beliefs; identify the emotions/bodily sensations. Note the cognitions and rate the percentage belief in them; and note also the accompanying behaviors, including the underlying and maintaining patterns of thought and behavior.

● SHELLY'S OLD WAYS OF BEING

OLD BEHAVIORS

Avoid observation whenever and wherever I can.

Make excuses to my supervisor before he observes a session or videotape.

Overprepare for sessions.

Avoid asking clients for feedback on the session.

OLD WAYS OF THINKING

If my work is seen by supervisors or colleagues, they'll see how useless I am. 85%

My clients see right through me. 80%

I'm no good as a therapist. 90%

I should be getting better results than I am. 100%

I should give up. 80%

EMOTIONS

Anxiety   Guilt   Fear   Self-doubt

Tension   Pain in pit of stomach

BODILY SENSATIONS

OLD UNDERLYING PATTERNS

Selective Attention—I focus on everything I do wrong, and don't pay any attention to the things I do well and this strengthens my belief that I'm really useless.

Rumination—When I feel a session doesn't go well, I go over and over it in my mind, beating myself up and dwelling on small mistakes.

Safety Behaviors—I overprepare for all my sessions trying to be ready for any contingency but I never learn what would happen if I didn't do this.

Worry—I'm always worrying about what my supervisor will think of me in an attempt to avoid potential criticism. This makes me appear stilted in supervision.

Avoidance—I avoid observation wherever possible to prevent my uselessness being seen. I don't get any direct feedback as a result.

ENVIRONMENT

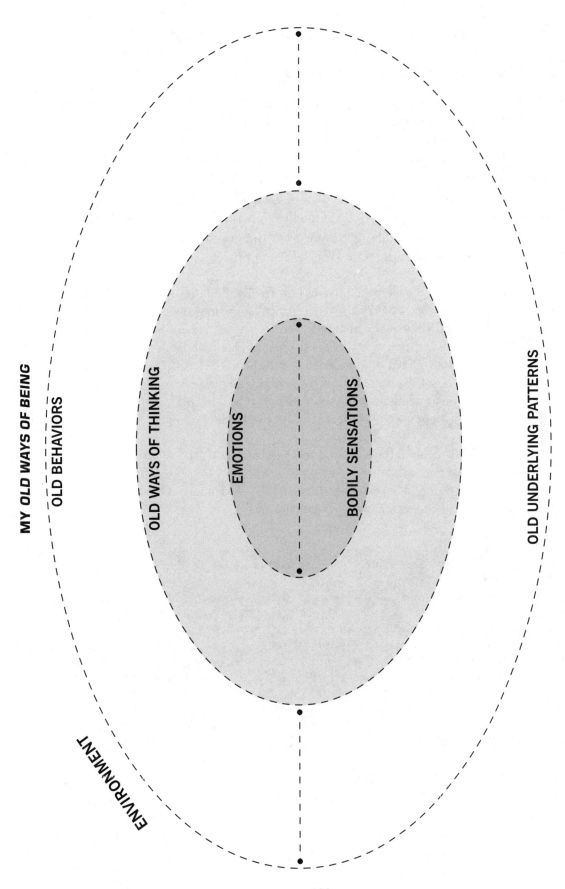

MY OLD WAYS OF BEING

OLD BEHAVIORS

OLD WAYS OF THINKING

EMOTIONS

BODILY SENSATIONS

OLD UNDERLYING PATTERNS

ENVIRONMENT

✍ **EXERCISE.** Establishing My *New Ways of Being*

Now it's time to create your *New Ways of Being*. Take a few minutes and find a quiet space to do an imagery exercise. This will be a bit like the imagery work you did for your goals, but adding in a bit more detail.

You might normally take two or three sessions to do this with clients, so give yourself enough time to "feel your way" into your *New Ways of Being*, and to note some of its features. Then go back and notice some more elements of the new ways. Before you do this exercise, take a moment to see what Shelly wrote on her *New Ways of Being* disk (page 195), and to review how she got there from the description below. Shelly used imagery. Imagery is central to the *New Ways of Being* process.

Shelly imagined herself as she would like to be—feeling, thinking, and doing things in exactly the way that she would want to. In particular, she imagined how she would feel in her body and emotionally, if things were going really well. She brought to mind her strengths (identified in Module 2) to underpin her *New Ways of Being*, and included these, along with her new underlying patterns, at the base of the disk. Then she identified the new behaviors and new ways of thinking, which would flow from her strengths and new underlying patterns. Notice that she rated her belief in her new ways of thinking, not just once but twice. She gave two kinds of rating:

- A "gut-level" belief rating—"how I feel inside (even if I know rationally it is probably not that bad)."
- A "rational-mind" belief rating (in parentheses)—"what my rational mind tells me is more in line with how things actually are."

> **The Key Question Is: "How Would I Like to Be?"**
>
> *Imagine yourself being exactly as you would like to be in the situations that have been a problem, even if right now it is hard to believe that you could feel or act in this way. See yourself clearly in one of these situations, but feeling exactly as you would like to feel, behaving in exactly the way that you would like to be behaving, thinking in exactly the way that you would like to be thinking about yourself and the situation. How do you want to be feeling? Do you notice any particular place in your body that you feel this? What do you see yourself doing? How does that feel? How does it feel to feel this way in your body? What personal strengths are you bringing to the situation? Feel these in your body too. What thoughts and images are you having: about you and about the situation? How is what you see yourself doing different from before? What new underlying patterns of thought and behavior are you incorporating into your repertoire?*

Once you've completed the whole disk on page 196, go back to the new ways of thinking and rate your belief in these new ideas. You may notice a difference between how it feels inside at gut level ("I'm useless." 100%) and how you would rate yourself if you think really rationally about it ("I'm useless." 50%). First tune in to "how it feels at a gut level" and put in this rating. Then add a "rational-mind" rating in parentheses.

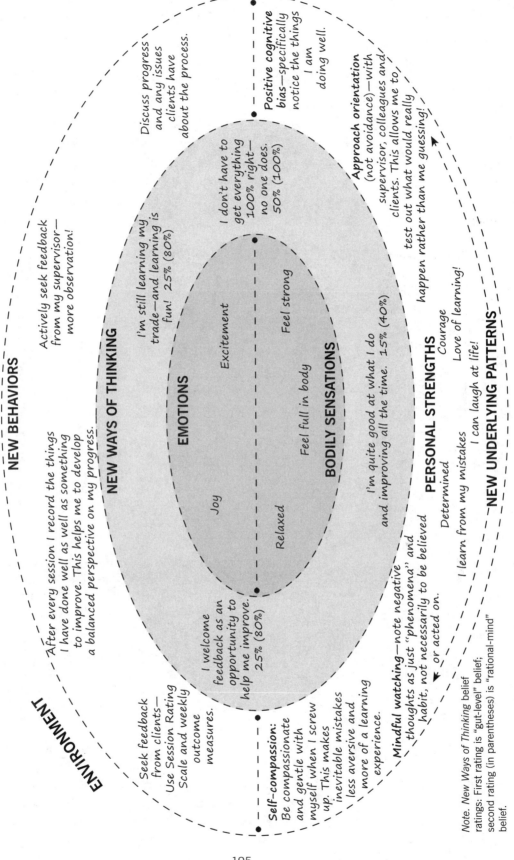

SHELLY'S NEW WAYS OF BEING

NEW BEHAVIORS

Actively seek feedback from my supervisor—more observation!

After every session I record the things I have done well as well as something to improve. This helps me to develop a balanced perspective on my progress.

Discuss progress and any issues clients have about the process.

NEW WAYS OF THINKING

I'm still learning my trade—and learning is fun! 25% (80%)

I don't have to get everything 100% right—no one does. 50% (100%)

Positive cognitive bias—specifically notice the things I am doing well.

Approach orientation (not avoidance)—with supervisor, colleagues and clients. This allows me to test out what would really happen rather than me guessing!

EMOTIONS

Excitement

Joy

Relaxed

Feel strong

Feel full in body

BODILY SENSATIONS

I'm quite good at what I do and improving all the time. 15% (40%)

PERSONAL STRENGTHS

Courage

Determined

Love of learning!

I can laugh at life!

I learn from my mistakes

NEW UNDERLYING PATTERNS

Mindful watching—note negative thoughts as just "phenomena" and habit, not necessarily to be believed or acted on.

Self-compassion: Be compassionate and gentle with myself when I screw up. This makes inevitable mistakes less aversive and more of a learning experience.

I welcome feedback as an opportunity to help me improve. 25% (80%)

Seek feedback from clients—Use Session Rating Scale and weekly outcome measures.

ENVIRONMENT

Note. New Ways of Thinking belief ratings: First rating is "gut-level" belief; second rating (in parentheses) is "rational-mind" belief.

195

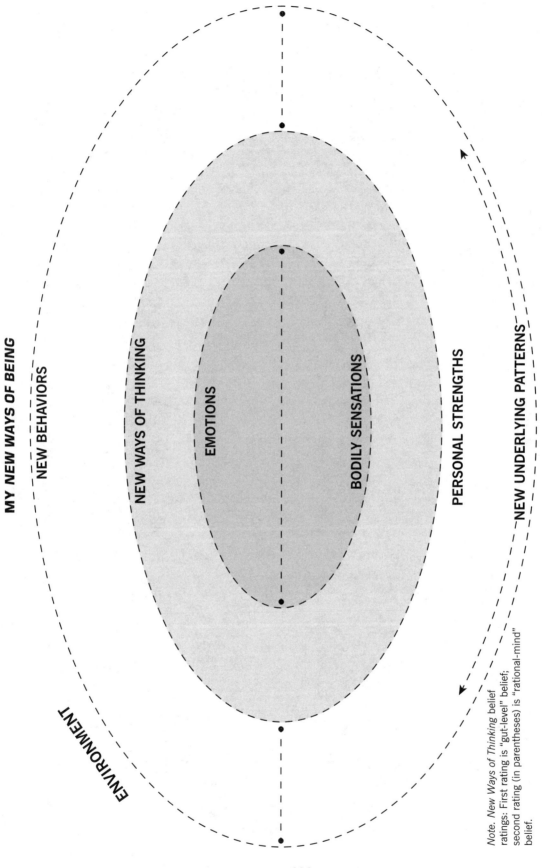

MY NEW WAYS OF BEING

NEW BEHAVIORS

NEW WAYS OF THINKING

EMOTIONS

BODILY SENSATIONS

PERSONAL STRENGTHS

NEW UNDERLYING PATTERNS

ENVIRONMENT

Note. New Ways of Thinking belief ratings: First rating is "gut-level" belief; second rating (in parentheses) is "rational-mind" belief.

You may find that at first you do not have much belief in the new ways of thinking, or confidence in the new patterns of behavior. There are a number of strategies that we can use to build belief and confidence. Here we introduce the *New Ways of Being* Record Book. In the next modules we shall introduce a number of other ways to strengthen new beliefs.

The *New Ways of Being* Record Book is based on the premise that the negative cognitive biases of our *Old Ways of Being* mean that we habitually pay attention to information that reinforces our *Old Ways of Being*; we systematically discount, ignore, distort, minimize, or do not notice information that might support an alternative, more positive *Way of Being*. For instance, in Shelly's case, she takes no notice of the fact that many of her clients are making good progress; that they regularly attend sessions; and that the feedback she has had from her supervisor has been almost wholly positive.

The *New Ways of Being* Record Book is designed to establish evidence to support the *New Ways of Being*. As *New Ways of Being* may take some time to establish and stabilize, the *New Ways of Being* Record Book should be used on a daily basis in the first weeks. We suggest that you use it regularly, preferably daily, over the period of the remaining modules. For more intransigent *Old Ways of Being*, clients may need to use the Record Book over some months. The idea of the *New Ways of Being* Record Book is to be constantly on the lookout for experiences that support the *News Ways of Being* that you have previously not noticed because of the negative bias (i.e., the idea is to catch yourself doing little things well to "build muscle" for the *New Ways of Being*).

To use the *New Ways of Being* Record Book, there are two preparatory tasks:

1. To develop a *News Ways of Being* summary statement that encapsulates key elements of your *New Ways of Being* (rather like the summary problem statement in Module 2)
2. To determine what kinds of behaviors, ways of thinking, demonstrations of personal strengths, or bodily feelings and emotions could be evidence that you are acting from your *New Ways of Being*.

These tasks are addressed in the Record Book preparation worksheet.

 EXAMPLE. Shelly's Record Book Preparation Worksheet

First we will look at Shelly's *New Ways of Being* Record Book preparation worksheet on page 198.

SHELLY'S RECORD BOOK PREPARATION WORKSHEET

My *New Ways of Being* summary statement
I'm looking to keep improving my skills all the time. I look out for what I do well in order to build my confidence. I purposely seek feedback from my supervisor and clients as I know this is the way that I'll learn most quickly— even if it's painful at times. I recognize that like anyone learning a trade, I'm bound to make mistakes. Everyone does! I'm not beating myself up for my mistakes. If I get negative, I note my thoughts, I am compassionate and gentle with myself recognizing that I am just learning. And then I refocus on all the things I am doing well.

Examples of the kinds of behaviors and ways of thinking and being (including my personal strengths) that demonstrate that I am acting from my *New Ways of Being* and will help me maintain these over time.
Recording therapy sessions (even if part of me doesn't want to!)   *Seeking feedback from my supervisor*   *Routinely getting feedback from clients, including satisfaction ratings (note to myself—use the Session Rating Scale)*   *Note when my clients are improving—and give myself a pat on the back*   *Moving on from negative feelings about myself more quickly*   *Routinely noting things I am doing well (after every session)*   *Congratulating myself for noting things I can improve on. Recognize that noting things down is a way to improve as a therapist.*   *Not beating myself up about things I am not doing well*   *Having a positive attitude to my client work*   *Looking forward to supervision sessions!*

 EXERCISE. My Record Book Preparation Worksheet

Now it is your turn to use the Preparation Worksheet on page 199 for the *New Ways of Being* Record Book

MY RECORD BOOK PREPARATION WORKSHEET

My *New Ways of Being* summary statement
Examples of the kinds of behaviors and ways of thinking and being (including my personal strengths) that demonstrate that I am acting from my *New Ways of Being* and will help me maintain these over time.

Using the *New Ways of Being* Record Book

To build "muscle" for the *New Ways of Being*, the Record Book is best used on a regular basis for a few weeks or sometimes months. Although data are lacking, our suggestion would be to note one to five examples of *New Ways of Being* every day in the Record Book for at least a month, and then to continue as needed. The *New Ways of Being* Record Book is included in this module and the remaining modules of the SP/SR workbook so that you can judge the value of repeated "muscle building" for yourself. A simple notebook or diary with each day demarcated is an ideal Record Book. Alternatively, you could use a notebook function in your mobile phone as a simple way to carry your Record Book around with you.

 EXAMPLE: Shelly's *New Ways of Being* Record Book

The box below shows what Shelly wrote in the first two days of her Record Book:

Examples of *My New Ways of Being*: Monday

1. I asked client MF for feedback.

2. I asked client MM for feedback and gave her a Session Rating Scale to complete. We then discussed her ratings. Great that she thought the session had really worked for her!

3. I asked client AH for feedback and gave her a Session Rating Scale to complete. We discussed her ratings. She told me that the session had been alright, but she doesn't feel she is making progress. I initially felt devastated. Then I remembered my New Ways of Being—of course, this is an opportunity to learn! I must ask her next time at the start of the session what she means by progress, what it would look like, and discuss how we might get there, what we might do differently. Maybe feedback is a good idea!

4. I have all these reports to do. I got really down on myself—until I remembered not to drown in my negative states—to do my mindful watching. That was actually helpful.

Examples of My *New Ways of Being*: Tuesday

1. Supervision—wow, this was so different! John said I'd done a good case formulation. He also thought I'd gone about setting up the behavioral experiment pretty well. Hey, I'm doing some things right—and noting the positive feedback from John, instead of thinking I just got lucky.

2. Supervision again . . . instead of trying to hide my feelings of inadequacy when working with client AH, I went for it and told John how I feel, what's happening in therapy, and about my stuckness. He actually complimented me for talking about my feelings, and then told me that he has often felt like that with clients! It was actually a great conversation, and I got some really useful ideas.

3. I did well in DW's session! He got the idea that his thinking really does influence how he feels, which is the first time he's really "got it."

---

4. GB is improving—BAI down 5 points since last week. I must be doing something right—well, actually she told me that "doing that funny imagery thing" made a big difference!

5. EH's session—not so good. No improvement. So stuck. Felt hopeless . . . No, that's okay, I'll take it to the next supervision session. It's an opportunity to learn . . . Well, I'm not quite over the feeling yet, but at least I can see that I can learn from this, rather than feel ashamed. And I'm going to be gentle with myself this evening and enjoy the concert—and damn well ensure I forget about the session!

 EXERCISE. My *New Ways of Being* Record Book

Create or buy a suitable Record Book, or use a smartphone, and start recording examples of your *New Ways of Being* on a daily basis over the next month. Mark off the days. Give yourself cues and reminders (e.g., using your mobile alarm) to remember to note the examples.

 Self-Reflective Questions

How easy or difficult was it to construct your *New Ways of Being*? How did this compare with mapping your *Old Ways of Being*? Was there any difference in how you felt inside while mapping the *Old Ways of Being* and constructing the *New Ways of Being*?

_____

_____

_____

_____

_____

_____

_____

_____

_____

_____

_____

_____

_____

How did you go with using imagery to construct your *New Ways of Being*? Is there anything else you could have done to construct the *New Ways of Being*?

_____

_____

_____

_____

_____

_____

_____

_____

_____

_____

_____

_____

_____

What are the implications for your clinical practice of your experience of establishing your *News Way of Being*?

_____

_____

_____

_____

_____

_____

_____

_____

_____

_____

_____

_____

_____

When doing belief ratings for your *New Ways of Being*, were there differences between the "gut-feeling" ratings and the "rational-mind" ratings? What sense do you make of this? How relevant is this for clients? How might you bring this distinction into your clinical practice?

_____

_____

_____

_____

_____

_____

_____

_____

_____

_____

_____

_____

What are you going to do to remind yourself to practice your *New Ways of Being* on a very regular basis?

_____

_____

_____

_____

_____

_____

_____

_____

_____

_____

_____

_____

_____

How easy or difficult has it been to find examples of your *New Ways of Being* using the Record Book? Are you noticing things that you would not previously have noticed? What do you make of this?

_____

_____

_____

_____

_____

_____

_____

_____

_____

_____

_____

_____

_____

_____

If you were to tell a colleague what you had gained from this module, what would you say?

_____

_____

_____

_____

_____

_____

_____

_____

_____

_____

_____

_____

_____

_____

_____

Embodying *New Ways of Being*

> I could imagine my story very well—I was there. . . . It helped me realize I may have been overlooking a lot of my *New Ways of Being*. . . . I won't forget it in a hurry. I feel it has served its purpose in helping me keep future focused—instead of looking back at evidence of what I am not, I will look forward for evidence of what I am.
>
> —SP/SR participant

In Module 9 you established your *New Ways of Being*, and set up the *New Ways of Being* Record Book to record examples of your *New Ways of Being* in action. The next two modules use a variety of strategies to strengthen the *New Ways of Being*. In this module, we use narrative, imagery, and body-oriented strategies, derived from the strengths-based work of Korrelboom and colleagues' COMET (**C**ompetitive **Me**mory **T**raining). In Module 11, we continue to build the *New Ways of Being* using behavioral experiments. We shall also be continuing with the *New Ways of Being* Record Book over the next weeks.

For this module, we suggest you do the exercises regularly over a number of sessions, so you may need to allow more time for this module. Developing *New Ways of Being* is about "building the muscle" of the new skills. Building the muscle takes time and practice like any physical fitness training, so the homework assignments designed to facilitate this are part of the module. The module is comprised of several distinct phases that you might choose to do at different times.

First, we review the *New Ways of Being* Record Book so far. As you will recall, we set this up as homework to be done on a daily basis.

✍🏻 EXERCISE. *New Ways of Being* Record Book Review

How has it been using the *New Ways of Being* Record Book to date? How much were you able to use it? Has there been an impact on your "gut-level" beliefs? How many times did you record examples? Used daily? Missed some days? Completely forgot about it or did not do it for some other reason? Record your responses in the form on page 208.

NEW WAYS OF BEING RECORD BOOK REVIEW

1. What has been the impact of the *New Ways of Being* Record Book?	
2. How much have you used the *New Ways of Being* Record Book since Module 9?	Number of days: Number of entries per day:
3. What (if anything) got in the way? If anything did get in the way, go back to Module 6—the *Reasons for Not Completing SP/SR Assignments* exercise. Check which of these might be relevant.	
4. If necessary, problem-solve how you might build the *New Ways of Being* Record Book into your daily routine in the next weeks. Use the problem-solving worksheet in Module 6 as a basis (e.g., define problem; brainstorm options, strengths, and weaknesses; solution selection; implementation planning; possible problems; how to overcome these problems).	

Typically, *Old (Unhelpful) Ways of Being* have a strong negative cognitive bias, making memories of past occasions of anxiety or failure highly accessible, and memories of past occasions of success relatively inaccessible. Kees Korrelboom and colleagues suggest that one of the ways to strengthen *New Ways of Being* is to search for and retrieve memories of past occasions in which we have displayed positive qualities in similar or related situations. We can then replay or reexperience those memories so that they become more salient for us. The strategies below are derived from Korrelboom's COMET training. COMET stands for **Co**mpetitive **Me**mory **T**raining, indicating that the purpose of the COMET intervention is to increase access to the positive memories (see Chapter 2 for the cognitive science rationale for COMET, derived from Chris Brewin's retrieval competition model).

Stories Where *New Ways of Being* Qualities Have Been in Evidence

The first of the COMET exercises involves writing a narrative about two occasions in which the *New Ways of Being* qualities were in evidence. These might be situations, similar to the current problem area, where the client shows positive qualities (e.g., persistence in a previous work situation); or other situations where similar types of qualities were evident (e.g., persistence at school, or persistence in completing a challenging 4-day walk). The exercise finishes with a summary of the positive qualities displayed.

 EXAMPLE: Shelly's Persistence at School in the Face of Adversity

Below is one of Shelly's stories, where her *New Ways of Being* qualities were in evidence. It comes from her schooldays:

Story 1

When I was 10, I was sick for 6 months with a "mystery illness" that later turned out to be a chronic fatigue-type virus. I missed over half a year at school. I didn't get to see my friends, and when I went back to school I felt like a bit of an outcast. I went into a class with a different bunch of kids who didn't seem to like me much. I remember going home and saying I wanted to stop going to school. I'd had it. But Mom and Dad insisted I went back. I really lacked confidence, I felt like I'd never catch up, that I'd always be struggling. That must have gone on for the next 3 months. But the turning point was that day when Mrs. Hawton took me to one side at the morning break, and sat me down on the wall by the sports field, and asked me how I was going. I told her the truth. I think she knew already. And she was so kind. She offered to give me extra time at the end of the school day—in the end, we only did this twice—and somehow her kindness made all the difference. From that moment, I got determined and decided I could do it. I caught up quickly. Within 2 or 3 weeks, I felt I was on top of things. Within 6 weeks, I was right up with the class, and after then I just flew for the rest of the year! It was probably my best year at school in the end.

What Does This Story Say about Me? And about My Positive Qualities?

I can show incredible determination and do very well when I get fired up. It seems to really help if I talk with someone and feel their support. Feeling the support seems to be enough until my own determination and persistence take over.

 EXERCISE. Stories Where *New Ways of Being* Qualities Have Been in Evidence

Recall two stories from the past where you demonstrated elements of your *New Ways of Being*. These might be situations, similar to the current problem area, where you have displayed positive qualities or other circumstances where similar types of qualities were evident. Describe the situations in as much detail as you can, elaborating on the qualities you displayed. In the summary sentence at the end of the stories note what the stories say about you and your qualities.

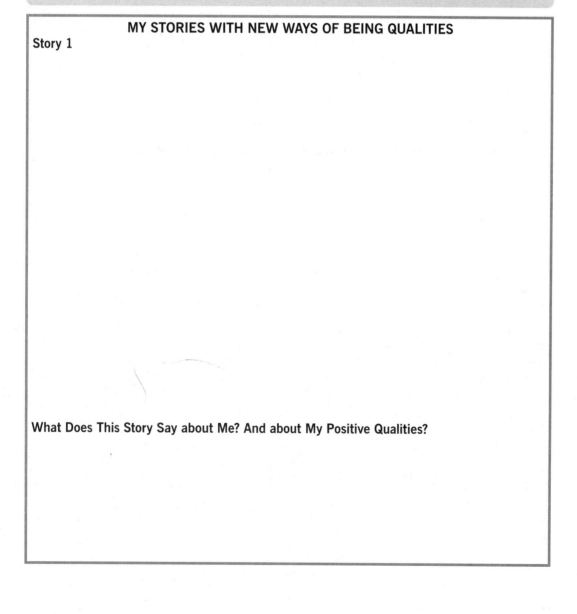

MY STORIES WITH NEW WAYS OF BEING QUALITIES

Story 1

What Does This Story Say about Me? And about My Positive Qualities?

Story 2

What Does This Story Say about Me? And about My Positive Qualities?

✍ **EXERCISE.** Reexperiencing the Story(ies) in Imagination

Which of these stories is the most convincing demonstration of the *New Ways of Being*? Read the stories again carefully.

> Take a few minutes of quiet time and use imagery to reexperience one or both stories: close your eyes, experience yourself being back in the situation, going through it again in slow motion in your mind. Notice your bodily sensations, your emotions, your actions from moment to moment as you focus in particular on the time period in which you displayed the positive qualities to greatest effect.
>
> If you have the time, take your second story, and go through a similar process.

REEXPERIENCING THE STORY(IES) IN IMAGINATION

What was your experience? What did you notice in your body and emotions? How did you feel afterward?

Adding Music and Body Movement
to the Story You Have Been Imagining

Research suggests that focusing on how we are feeling in our body and listening to uplifting music can heighten emotion and positive experience. The next exercise adds music and body movement to narrative and imagery. First, select a piece of music that for you symbolizes all the positive qualities that you showed in the story(ies). In the exercise, you will be asked to move your body in a way that captures the positive qualities you are experiencing in the situation and to do this accompanied by your chosen music.

 EXAMPLE: Shelly Added Music and Body Movement

First Shelly selected one of her favorite pieces of music that, for her, symbolized strength, power, and determination. Then when she put movement to it, she noticed how tall she felt as she walked, and how her shoulders and back felt much stronger. She felt strong and refreshed—ready to take on the world!

EXERCISE. Adding Music and Body Movement to the Story You Have
Been Imagining

Experience your story in your body by using movement, music, and imagery. In particular, feel the most important qualities that came out of your story. Your movement should symbolize how you feel when you experience these qualities. Bring to mind an image of yourself in the middle of the story, expressing these qualities. Play the music, and at the same time move your body (e.g., walk, express with hands, arms, legs, face). Notice how you feel. Keep doing so for a few minutes, noticing how you feel in yourself, body and mind. Repeat the exercise at least four times in the next week.

ADDING MUSIC AND BODY MOVEMENT TO MY STORY

What was your experience?

Your *New Ways of Being* will almost inevitably encounter problems when challenged by difficult situations. To anticipate and address them, we can identify particular issues that may be a problem, and develop strategies to deal with them.

 EXERCISE. Anticipating Potential Problems

What situations do you anticipate will cause problems for your *New Ways of Being*? This might include your own emotional, cognitive, or behavioral responses; the behavior of others; or factors to do with the environment (e.g., home or workplace rules or procedures). Note these situations on page 213:

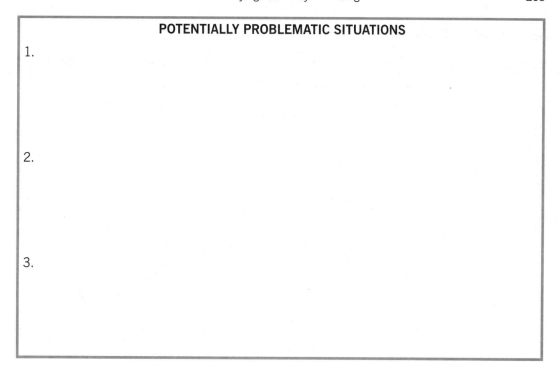

POTENTIALLY PROBLEMATIC SITUATIONS

1.

2.

3.

Ideas or Rules to Address Potential Problems

We use problem-solving strategies (as in Module 6) to address potential problems. An effective way to address *New Ways of Being* problems is to create specific rules to counter them, as in Module 7 on underlying assumptions and rules for living. These rules may take the form of *If . . .* [name problem], *then . . .* [corrective strategy] statements.

 EXAMPLE: Shelly's New Rule to Address a Potential Problem

One of Shelly's problematic situations was caused by her clients failing to improve. Using a problem-solving approach, she brainstormed various options:

- *Don't automatically attribute their lack of improvement to my lack of skill, there are many other possibilities that I can't control.*
- *Many clients don't improve during therapy, that's reality.*
- *Ask them to list the factors to which they attribute the lack of improvement.*
- *Discuss options with them.*
- *Discuss these cases with my supervisor.*

The rule that she developed was: *If* my client isn't improving, *then* there are many possible reasons, only one of which is a lack of skill on my part. Don't jump to premature conclusions before first carefully investigating the reasons!

EXERCISE. My New Rule(s) to Address Potential Problems

Create one or more rules for yourself to address potential problems, using the *If* . . . [problem], *Then* . . . [corrective strategy] format.

MY NEW RULES

1.

2.

3.

4.

 EXERCISE. Homework to Strengthen My *New Ways of Being*

Building *New Ways of Being* muscle involves regular (daily) practice—imaginal and behavioral—experimentation, and feedback, and then making adjustments where necessary. Homework is therefore an essential part of *New Ways of Being* work to establish new ways of thinking, patterns, emotions, and behaviors. To gain an experience of building *New Ways of Being*, below are two homework exercises to practice over the coming weeks. You may want to use Post-it notes and/or diary reminders to help you remember to practice and record your experiences each day.

Using movement and music, practice imagining yourself implementing new rules, patterns, and behaviors to address potentially problematic situations on at least 4 days over the next week. Note the impact in the *New Ways of Being* Imagery Homework Practice record sheet on page 215.

Also, continue your *New Ways of Being* Record Book on a daily basis. Note the impact.

NEW WAYS OF BEING IMAGERY HOMEWORK PRACTICE

Day 1 Impact

Day 2 Impact

Day 3 Impact

Day 4 Impact

Self-Reflective Questions

What was it like finding stories from the past where the *New Ways of Being* qualities were displayed? How easy or hard were they to write about? What did you experience bodily, emotionally, and cognitively as you wrote about them? How easy or hard were they to imagine? What was the impact?

_____

_____

_____

_____

_____

_____

_____

_____

_____

_____

_____

How might the ease or difficulty you experienced in retrieving the stories relate to clients' experiences? How would your own experience assist you in your work with clients?

_____

_____

_____

_____

_____

_____

_____

_____

_____

_____

_____

_____

Did the movement and music make a difference to how you felt? Did you continue to practice? How do you think this might translate to your clinical practice?

_____

_____

_____

_____

_____

_____

_____

_____

_____

_____

_____

_____

_____

You may not have previously come across the approach to building *New Ways of Being* used in this module. How comfortably does this new approach fit with how you usually use your CBT skills? What thoughts and feelings come up for you when you imagine using this intervention with clients? Do these thoughts and feelings mirror any of your other reactions over the course of the workbook? If so, are there any links you can make?

_____

_____

_____

_____

_____

_____

_____

_____

_____

_____

_____

_____

_____

_____

With regard to your belief and confidence in your *New Ways of Being*, are you experiencing any conflict between how much you believe your *New Ways of Being* rationally, and how much you believe it in your "heart" or "gut"? You have contrasted "head" and "heart" before. Are you experiencing any change regarding these two ways of processing information about yourself?

_____

_____

_____

_____

_____

_____

_____

_____

_____

_____

_____

_____

_____

What was the hardest thing to do? Did anything come particularly easily? If so, can you explain? What parts of this module really stand out for you that you would like to remember?

_____

_____

_____

_____

_____

_____

_____

_____

_____

_____

_____

_____

_____

MODULE 11

Using Behavioral Experiments to Test and Strengthen *New Ways of Being*

The only difficulty I had choosing an experiment was that I felt I had so much choice. This was definitely noteworthy as I feel that I would have really struggled with this 6 months ago, due to my (old) tendency to avoid. My *Old Ways of Being* would have certainly got in the way—don't do that, you'll look foolish, they won't like you, you'll get hurt. Ha, silly *Old Ways of Being*.

—SP/SR participant

In Module 8 we discussed the different types of behavioral experiments and their purpose. You tested out an unhelpful assumption related to your *Old Ways of Being* and compared this with a new alternative assumption. In Modules 9 and 10, we introduced the idea of developing and strengthening *New Ways of Being* using techniques ranging from imagery to the *New Ways of Being* Record Book. In this module you will be creating another behavioral experiment, but this time you will be aiming to build evidence for a new, helpful, work- or personal-related assumption specifically designed to strengthen your *New Ways of Being*. However, before doing so, let us just check on how you have been going with the *New Ways of Being* Record Book and the embodying exercises you practiced in Module 10.

✍ **EXERCISE. Reviewing the *New Ways* Record Book and the Embodying Exercises**

Complete the form on page 221.

NEW WAYS OF BEING RECORD BOOK
AND EMBODYING EXERCISES REVIEW

New Ways of Being Record Book:
Have you been able to record more examples of *New Ways of Being* since Module 10? If so, what has been the impact?
If not, what has got in the way, and what might you do to get back on track?

Embodying exercises:
Have you been able to put any of the embodying exercises (narratives, imagery, movement, and music) into practice? How has this gone?
If you have been unable or unwilling to, what has got in the way? Is there a strategy you can put in place to address this? (If anything did get in the way, perhaps go back to Module 6— the *Reasons for Not Completing Weekly Activities* exercise. Check which of these might be relevant.)

Identifying a *New Ways of Being* Assumption for the Behavioral Experiment

As you have seen in Module 8, to create a behavioral experiment we need to identify a specific assumption or belief that can be tested by a specific experiment or series of experiments. Usually when people are testing a negative assumption or noting whether a feared catastrophe does actually take place, questioning can reveal a clear thought (verbal or image-based) that can be directly tested (e.g., "I will be laughed at," "I will fail," "I will be rejected"). However, when we are in our *Old Ways of Being* mind-set testing a negative assumption, it is often hard to make specific *positive* predictions.

As you are already in the process of developing your *New Ways of Being*, you may be approaching the next behavioral experiment with a stronger belief in a new assumption, or set of assumptions, than in the previous behavioral experiment in Module 8. However, there may still be a gap between your intellectual and your gut- level beliefs. This experiment is a chance to "road-test" a new assumption and gain some experiential understanding of how it may "fit" in practice. You can discover what happens when you practice a new way of behaving associated with your *New Ways of Being*. How does it feel? How do people react? What can you learn? Does the assumption need to be tweaked or adjusted?

 EXAMPLE: Jayashri's *New Ways of Being* Assumption

In the early modules of the SP/SR workbook, Jayashri identified that she tended to be very critical of anything she perceived as a fault, and struggled to be compassionate with herself. She identified an assumption "If I am compassionate with myself, it will lead to an acceptance of failure, laziness, and low standards." At some level she believed that self-criticism was useful and the only way to improve. During Modules 7–10, Jayashri began to realize that it might be helpful to integrate self-compassion into her *New Ways of Being*. She knew that she could be very compassionate with others (e.g., toward her younger sister), but realized that she had a much harsher attitude toward herself, which was sabotaging her confidence. Her new assumption to be tested was "If I show self-compassion and acceptance toward myself following a mistake, it will make it easier to change and improve." She already had some evidence for this idea from her earlier experiments but thought that a direct test of the assumption might give her a real "gut-level" experience, which might start to cement a new way of thinking.

 EXERCISE. Creating My *New Ways of Being* Assumption

To identify an assumption that you would like to test, it may be helpful now to spend some time refocusing on your work in Modules 9 and 10 to get yourself "into the zone." Fully imagine your *New Ways of Being*; see if you can experience a felt sense of what it would be like to think and feel and behave in this way. Once immersed in your *New Ways of Being*, use the experience to identify a helpful assumption that can be tested by a behavioral experiment. Alternatively, you may want to use the new assumption from Module 8, and create another experiment to build more evidence for it.

My *New Ways of Being* assumption to be tested is:

Planning the Behavioral Experiment

The *New Ways of Being* Behavioral Experiment Record Sheet is very similar to the planning worksheet to compare old and new assumptions in Module 8, except that there is no focus on any "old assumption." The purpose is to build evidence for the new assumption, derived from the *New Ways of Being*. As in Module 8, we identify and troubleshoot any potential problems, and then carry out the behavioral experiment and complete the review sheet. Following the experiment, we aim to allow the outcome to really "sink in," then use the findings to generate clear follow-up actions.

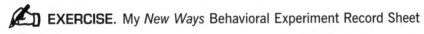 **EXERCISE.** My *New Ways* Behavioral Experiment Record Sheet

First look at Shelly's example on pages 224–225. Shelly decided to test her *New Ways of Being* in the context of a supervision session. Then complete your planning record sheet on pages 226–227 in as much detail as possible.

SHELLY'S NEW WAYS BEHAVIORAL EXPERIMENT RECORD SHEET (FIRST THREE COLUMNS)

Target cognition(s)	Experiment	Prediction(s)	Outcome	What I learned
What are some of your New Ways of Thinking? What would be a helpful New Ways assumption to test? Rate belief in cognitions (0–100%) firstly as a "gut-level" belief rating, then with "rational-mind" rating in parentheses.	Design an experiment to test out the New Ways idea. Which of your strengths and New Ways of Being might be useful here?	What do you predict will happen from your New Ways perspective? How likely do you think this is ("gut-level" and "rational-mind" ratings)? (0–100%)	What actually happened? What did you observe about yourself (behavior, thoughts, feelings, bodily sensations)? About your environment, about other people? Any difficulties? What did you do about them? How does the outcome fit with your predictions?	How much do you now believe your New Ways assumption (0–100%)? What have you learned about any safety behaviors? Will you be dropping them? What are the practical implications? Does your New Ways assumption need to be modified? If so, what might the modified version be? **Belief Ratings:** **New Ways Assumption** ___% (___%)
New Ways of Thinking I don't have to get everything 100% right—no one does. I'm still learning my trade—and learning is fun. I'm quite good at what I do and improving all the time.	During the next week I will take a case to supervision where I've got stuck and be honest about not knowing what to do. I won't hide from this or pretend that everything is going well.	My supervisor will appreciate my honesty and will help me learn—that's what he is there for. I will feel anxious and vulnerable but will benefit overall. 30% (70%)		
New Ways Assumption If I admit to my supervisor that I don't know what to do with a client, he will support me and I will learn from the experience. 10% (85%)				

224

Troubleshooting potential problems

What old ways of behaving might you fall into?

I might try and avoid recording a session by not asking clients or even pretend that my video camera is broken. I might try and divert supervision into a discussion around risk to avoid showing the recording.

Which of your strengths and *New Ways of Being* might be useful here?

I am determined and I stick to things. I know what I need to do here and I need to use my "stickability"! I now have real insight into my patterns and know what I need to do differently. I have shown myself that I can make big changes before (e.g., when I lost lots of weight).

How will you use these identified personal strengths and new ways to prevent yourself doing this? What will you do instead?

I will first notice the thoughts telling me to avoid recording. I will remind myself of some of the images I have been working on at times when I have been brave and gone against my old ways of thinking and behaving. I will feel the anxiety and let it remind me that I am doing something new and it's not something to be avoided.

What practical problems might get in the way?

My supervisor might cancel the session (he said he might have to give expert evidence in court) or my camera might have problems.

How will you deal with these?

I will test out my camera in advance and then ask as many clients as possible to ensure I am ready and know what I'm doing. If my supervisor has to cancel, then I will show the recording to a colleague for feedback.

MY NEW WAYS BEHAVIORAL EXPERIMENT RECORD SHEET

Target cognition(s)	Experiment	Prediction(s)	Outcome	What I learned
What are some of your New Ways of Thinking? What would be a helpful New Ways assumption to test? Rate belief in cognitions (0–100%) firstly as a "gut-level" belief rating, then with "rational-mind" rating in parentheses.	Design an experiment to test out the New Ways idea. Which of your strengths and New Ways of Being might be useful here?	What do you predict will happen from your New Ways perspective? How likely do you think this is ("gut-level" and "rational-mind" ratings)? (0–100%)	What actually happened? What did you observe about yourself (behavior, thoughts, feelings, bodily sensations)? About your environment, about other people? Any difficulties? What did you do about them? How does the outcome fit with your predictions?	How much do you now believe your New Ways assumption (0–100%)? What have you learned about any safety behaviors? Will you be dropping them? What are the practical implications? Does your New Ways assumption need to be modified? If so, what might the modified version be?
New Ways of Thinking				**Belief Ratings:** *New Ways Assumption* ____ % (____ %)
New Ways Assumption				

226

Troubleshooting potential problems

What old ways of behaving might you fall into?

Which of your strengths and *New Ways of Being* might be useful here?

How will you use these identified personal strengths and new ways to prevent yourself doing this? What will you do instead?

What practical problems might get in the way?

How will you deal with these?

227

Outcome of the Behavioral Experiment

As in Module 8, the next step after completing a behavioral experiment is to take some time to think about what happened (and what did not happen) so that you can complete the fourth and fifth columns of your *New Ways* Behavioral Experiment Record Sheet on page 226. These two columns ask the kinds of questions that will help you to summarize the experience and to plan the next steps.

 EXERCISE. My *New Ways* Behavioral Experiment Review Worksheet

Now review what happened in your experiment by going back to your Behavioral Experiment Record Sheet on pages 226–227 and completing the last two columns, "Outcome" and "What I learned."

On page 229, you can see how Shelly made sense of her behavioral experiment.

SHELLY'S *NEW WAYS* BEHAVIORAL EXPERIMENT RECORD SHEET

Target cognition(s)	Experiment	Prediction(s)	Outcome	What I learned
What are some of your *New Ways of Thinking*? What would be a helpful *New Ways* assumption to test? Rate belief in cognitions (0–100%) firstly as a "gut-level" belief rating, then with "rational-mind" rating in parentheses.	Design an experiment to test out the *New Ways* idea. Which of your strengths and *New Ways of Being* might be useful here?	What do you predict will happen from your *New Ways* perspective? How likely do you think this is ("gut-level" and "rational-mind" ratings)? (0–100%)?	What actually happened? What did you observe about yourself (behavior, thoughts, feelings, bodily sensations? About your environment, about other people? Any difficulties? What did you do about them? How does the outcome fit with your predictions?	How much do you now believe your *New Ways* assumption (0–100%)? What have you learned about any safety behaviors? Will you be dropping them? What are the practical implications? Does your *New Ways* assumption need to be modified? If so, what might the modified version be?
New Ways of Thinking *I don't have to get everything 100% right—no one does.* *I'm still learning my trade—and learning is fun.* *I'm quite good at what I do and improving all the time.*	*During the next week I will take a case to supervision where I've got stuck and be honest about not knowing what to do. I won't hide from this or pretend that everything is going well.*	*My supervisor will appreciate my honesty and will help me learn—that's what he is there for. I will feel anxious and vulnerable but will benefit overall.* 30% (70%)	*I recorded loads of sessions and took them to supervision, admitting I was stuck! I felt quite anxious but all the preparatory work really helped and I kept reminding myself that I was trying to break the old ways of behaving and try something new. My supervisor was so helpful. He helped me to realize that I had learned more than I thought. Even the fact that he didn't laugh at me or suggest I resign was reassuring. I felt more confident at a gut level. This really strengthened my new belief and helped me reconsider my beliefs about others too.*	**Belief Ratings:** ***New Ways Assumption*** <u>90</u> % (100%) *I think I can widen this assumption. I realize that I worry about being found out in a wide range of situations. My new assumption needs to be more along the lines of "If I take risks and try new things, I may feel anxious but I won't automatically be judged. I should take more risks!"*
New Ways Assumption *If I admit to my supervisor that I don't know what to do with a client, he will support me and I will learn from the experience.* 10% (85%)			*No major difficulties or surprises. I had planned this experiment quite well and was more able to cope with blips (e.g., first client refused to be recorded) by reminding myself of the previous situations where I had pushed and challenged myself and how strong I had felt afterward.* *It completely supported my predictions around my new assumptions! It really cemented them at a gut level. Definitely made that shift—I wish I'd done it earlier.*	*At work I need to put myself in more anxiety-provoking situations, I need to remember that new situations are challenging but help me grow and learn. I have agreed to do some teaching next month and that brings up even more thoughts. No more old ways!*

Creating Follow-Up Experiments

As we saw in Module 8, it is often important to create follow-up experiments to embed *New Ways of Being.*

 EXAMPLE: Shelly's Follow-Up Experiments

Shelly realized that though the *New Ways* experiment with her supervisor had been successful, she might justifiably or unjustifiably be criticized by somebody in the future; and that it would be important that she could handle criticism without her self-esteem collapsing.

SHELLY'S FOLLOW-UP EXPERIMENTS: WHAT, WHERE, WITH WHOM?

There might be situations where I try new things and get them wrong . . . Part of me is still worried about being criticized but sooner or later I will be criticized! I need to test out my reactions and beliefs about criticism or making mistakes. I need to keep exposing myself to new situations outside my comfort zone, maybe even practice making some mistakes on purpose. I will start off small by giving someone in a store the wrong money—I can work up from there . . .

 EXERCISE. My Follow-Up Experiments

In the box below, create one or more behavioral experiments which will be potentially helpful to strengthen your *New Ways of Being.*

MY FOLLOW-UP EXPERIMENTS: WHAT, WHERE, WITH WHOM?

Creating a Summary Image, Metaphor, or Drawing

As a final exercise in this module, it can be very helpful to capture the *New Ways of Being* in one summary image, metaphor, or drawing: something that symbolizes your *New Ways of Being* that can be used on a day-to-day basis to cue you to embody your *New Ways*. It may be helpful to incorporate cultural icons into your image. The icons might make use of common cultural symbols or encapsulate qualities of one of your "heroes"—for example, embodying a Mandela-like willingness to collaborate without rancor with a person who may have done you wrong.

 EXAMPLE: Jayashri's Summary Image, Metaphor, or Drawing

> Jayashri downloaded a picture of a lotus flower from the Internet to remind her to be self-compassionate. She made several copies and put the picture on her desk, at the front of her diary, and in the therapy room.

 EXERCISE. My Summary Image, Metaphor, or Drawing

Take a few quiet minutes now to see if you can come up with an image, metaphor, or drawing that symbolizes your *New Ways of Being*. Make some notes, draw, or reproduce the image in the space below.

MY IMAGE/METAPHOR/DRAWING

You may well find that over the next week(s) you find an even more suitable image or metaphor. If you do, note this and practice using the new version. Create cues and reminders so that you can summon the image or metaphor many times a day to embed it into your being. Plan these now. What cues will you use?

+---+
| **CUES AND REMINDERS FOR MY IMAGE OR METAPHOR** |
| |
| |
| |
| |
| |
| |
| |
| |
| |
| |
| |
+---+

Self-Reflective Questions

What did you notice when you were planning your behavioral experiment to test out your *New Ways* assumption? (What were your emotions? Bodily sensations? Thoughts? Behaviors? Was there anything that surprised you?)

_____

_____

_____

_____

_____

_____

_____

_____

_____

_____

_____

_____

_____

Looking back on your behavioral experiment and trying to make sense of what actually happened, how does it feel? Thinking about your *New Ways* assumption, is there any mismatch between "head" and "gut" levels of belief?

_____

_____

_____

_____

_____

_____

_____

_____

_____

_____

_____

_____

When you bring to mind what happened in your *New Ways* experiment, can you identify anything that you learned about yourself either as a therapist or in your life outside work? Or maybe even something that applied across both?

_____

_____

_____

_____

_____

_____

_____

_____

_____

_____

_____

_____

How do you now understand the purpose of testing *New Ways* and *Old Ways* in your CBT practice?

_____

_____

_____

_____

_____

_____

_____

_____

_____

_____

_____

_____

_____

How did you go with creating an image, metaphor, or drawing to encapsulate your *New Ways of Being*? Was this useful? Was there anything that got in the way? If so, what might have helped?

_____

_____

_____

_____

_____

_____

_____

_____

_____

_____

_____

_____

_____

What have you learned during this module that feels important to remember?

_____

_____

_____

_____

_____

_____

_____

_____

_____

_____

_____

_____

Maintaining and Enhancing
New Ways of Being

I think the *New Ways of Being* Maintenance Plan itself will help to keep me on track. I have worried that I will get to the end of this, drop it, and forget everything—I really don't want to do this!!! So I'll type up my *New Ways of Being* Maintenance Plan, get it all nice and pretty, and keep it somewhere safe!
—SP/SR participant

A pivotal goal in CBT is to empower clients with both the skills and the belief that they can become their own therapist once therapy has ended. One way to do this is to focus on "relapse prevention" from the start of therapy—and of course, to emphasize relapse prevention as therapy draws to a close. In those final sessions, the therapist encourages the client to review the progress he or she has made toward understanding, managing, and overcoming the problems that brought him or her to therapy. Typically, client and therapist review the client's progress toward goals and identify the CBT skills that have proved valuable. Then they consider what obstacles to progress the client may face in the future, anticipate ways of coping with these obstacles, and focus on recognizing early warning signs in order to take preventative action. The endpoint of this process is usually a summary sheet, sometimes called a "blueprint," which clients take home to remind them about what to do to build on the progress they have made in therapy.

From the strengths-based perspective of *Experiencing CBT from the Inside Out*, the aim of the final sessions is not so much "relapse prevention," but rather "maintaining and enhancing *New Ways of Being*." We are looking to assist clients to consolidate and firmly establish the *New Ways of Being* in their lives, as you have been doing in this workbook, particularly in these latest modules.

This final module has two purposes. First, it takes you through a maintaining and enhancing *New Ways of Being* process similar to one you might use with clients. You will be reviewing your *New Ways of Being* self-formulation and belief ratings, and developing a personal "blueprint" that we have called "My *New Ways of Being* Maintenance Plan."

A second purpose of the module is to reflect on your experience of SP/SR for your professional development as a CBT therapist. The reason you have engaged with the workbook has been to "experience CBT from the inside out" using your "personal self" or "therapist self" (or probably both), and to reflect on what this means for your work with clients from a "therapist self" perspective. What has the experience been like? Has it been valuable? If so, how? Are there any implications for your future? How might you apply what you have learned through SP/SR to your continued development as a therapist and in your wider life? It may be that there are aspects of SP/SR practice that you would like to build into your professional (and/or personal) roles for the future.

 EXERCISE. Reviewing the PHQ-9 and GAD-7

As a first step, rerate yourself on the PHQ-9 and GAD-7, using the forms below and on page 239, just as you might typically ask a client to do at the end of therapy. If you have used any other questionnaires to monitor your progress, now is the time to rerate yourself on these as well.

PHQ-9: POST-SP/SR

Over the last 2 weeks, how often have you been bothered by the following problems?	Not at all	Several days	More than half the days	Nearly every day
1. Little interest or pleasure in doing things	0	1	2	3
2. Feeling down, depressed, or hopeless	0	1	2	3
3. Trouble falling or staying asleep, or sleeping too much	0	1	2	3
4. Feeling tired or having little energy	0	1	2	3
5. Poor appetite or overeating	0	1	2	3
6. Feeling bad about yourself—or that you are a failure or have let yourself or your family down	0	1	2	3
7. Trouble concentrating on things, such as reading the newspaper or watching television	0	1	2	3
8. Moving or speaking so slowly that other people could have noticed? Or the opposite—being so fidgety or restless that you have been moving around a lot more than usual	0	1	2	3
9. Thoughts that you would be better off dead or of hurting yourself in some way	0	1	2	3

You can calculate your total score on the PHQ-9 by adding each item.

0–4:	No indication of depression
5–9:	Indicative of mild depression
10–14:	Indicative of moderate depression
15–19:	Indicative of moderately severe depression
20–27:	Indicative of severe depression
	My score: _____

GAD-7: POST-SP/SR

Over the last 2 weeks, how often have you been bothered by the following problems?	Not at all	Several days	More than half the days	Nearly every day
1. Feeling nervous, anxious, or on edge	0	1	2	3
2. Not being able to stop or control worrying	0	1	2	3
3. Worrying too much about different things	0	1	2	3
4. Trouble relaxing	0	1	2	3
5. Being so restless that it is hard to sit still	0	1	2	3
6. Becoming easily annoyed or irritable	0	1	2	3
7. Feeling afraid as if something awful might happen	0	1	2	3

You can calculate your total score on the GAD-7 by adding each item.

Scores of:	
0–4:	No indication of anxiety
5–9:	Indicative of mild anxiety
10–14:	Indicative of moderate anxiety
15–21:	Indicative of severe anxiety
	My score: _____

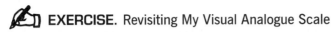 **EXERCISE.** Revisiting My Visual Analogue Scale

Review your initial challenging problem (Module 1). As a reminder, briefly summarize the problem area below. Rate your *current* level of distress now using the VAS that you developed in Module 1, and compare this with your previous score. Has there been a change? To what extent? What do you attribute this to?

MY VISUAL ANALOGUE SCALE

My Challenging Problem:

0% ————————————————	50% ————————————————	100%
Not present	Moderate	Most severe
0% Description	50% Description	100% Description

 EXERCISE. Reviewing My Goals

Look at Modules 2 and 6 and remind yourself of your goals and the progress you had made by Module 6. How are you doing now? Complete the form on page 241 to summarize your experience, and your next steps.

REVIEWING MY GOALS

	Goal 1	Goal 2
Comment on your progress with each goal. How did you go with the time frames you set for yourself? Were they as realistic and achievable as you originally thought? Were they measurable?		
What roadblocks were there (if any)? • Internal factors (e.g., your self-doubt, low motivation, old patterns of procrastination, self-criticism) • External factors over which you have some control (e.g., business, family demands) • External factors outside of your control		
What are your next steps?		

241

✍ EXERCISE. Reviewing My *Old Ways of Being/New Ways of Being*

My *Old Ways of Being* Self-Formulation

First, go back to Module 9 and review your *Old Ways of Being* self-formulation. How familiar does this seem? Has there been any change? If so, what have you noticed? Are you spending as much time in your *Old Ways of Being*, looking through these lenses? If not, what has changed? Write your reflections in the box below.

MY *OLD WAYS OF BEING*: WHAT DIFFERENCES HAVE I NOTICED?

My *New Ways of Being* Self-Formulation

Review your *New Ways of Being* disk in Module 9, or, better still, copy it into the *New Ways of Being* disk on page 243 to further embed the new ways. See if there is anything you would like to add—for instance, you may want to add the image or metaphor you developed in Module 11, or some strengths that you did not consider at the time.

Now review the new ways of thinking. Write the new ways of thinking from Module 9 into the *New Ways of Being* disk on page 243 and rerate these cognitions with "gut-level" and "rational-mind" ratings. Are there any differences from the ratings in Module 9? What are they? How much progress have you made? What has made the difference?

MY *NEW WAYS OF BEING*: WHAT DIFFERENCES HAVE I NOTICED?

MY NEW WAYS OF BEING

NEW BEHAVIORS

NEW WAYS OF THINKING

EMOTIONS

BODILY SENSATIONS

PERSONAL STRENGTHS

NEW UNDERLYING PATTERNS

ENVIRONMENT

Note. New Ways of Thinking belief ratings: First rating is "gut-level" belief; second rating (in parentheses) is "rational-mind" belief.

From *Experiencing CBT from the Inside Out: A Self-Practice/Self-Reflection Workbook for Therapists* by James Bennett-Levy, Richard Thwaites, Beverly Haarhoff, and Helen Perry. Copyright 2015 by The Guilford Press. Permission to photocopy this form is granted to purchasers of this book for personal use only (see copyright page for details). Purchasers can download this material from *www.guilford.com/bennett-levy-forms*.

My *New Ways of Being* Record Book

Have you been able to maintain the *New Ways of Being* Record Book? Has it made a difference? If so, how? If you have not been able to maintain it, what has got in the way? Were you able to address this problem in any way? What might have helped you to do so? What are the implications for clients?

MY *NEW WAYS OF BEING* RECORD BOOK: WHAT HAS BEEN ITS IMPACT?

My *New Ways* Narratives, Imagery, Music, and Body Movement (COMET Exercises)

Have you continued to reflect on the *New Ways of Being* stories that you wrote and imagined in Module 10? Have you been able to embed them so that they are more retrievable? Have you practiced using music and movement? Has this made a difference?

MY *NEW WAYS* NARRATIVES, IMAGERY, MUSIC, AND BODY MOVEMENT: HOW HELPFUL HAVE THEY BEEN?

My Behavioral Experiments

What has been the impact of the behavioral experiments? Have you found yourself creating other behavioral experiments, or thinking about your experience in a "behavioral experiment" kind of way? Has it been easy or difficult to design behavioral experiments, or to follow through with them?

MY BEHAVIORAL EXPERIMENTS: WHAT HAS BEEN THEIR IMPACT?

My Summary Imagery, Metaphor, or Drawing

Have you found the summary imagery, metaphor, or drawing at the end of Module 11 useful? Have you been able to bring it to mind at appropriate times? How often? What has enabled you to do so, or what has got in the way?

IMAGERY, METAPHORS, AND DRAWINGS: WHAT HAVE I NOTICED?

 EXERCISE. What Helped Me to Move from the *Old* to the *New Ways of Being*?

Look back over the workbook. Were there any self-practice exercises that were particularly useful in enabling you to move from *Old* to *New Ways of Being* (e.g., formulating using the five-part model including strengths and cultural factors, activity scheduling, using thought records, imagery, metaphor, behavioral experiments, body-oriented strategies, increasing access to positive memories, the *New Ways of Being* Record Book, or problem solving using your "new rules" developed to address potential problems)? Make a list of these below and circle the ones you want to remember to keep using for the future.

MY MOST USEFUL SELF-PRACTICE EXERCISES

Were there any examples of "aha" moments? What were they?

✍ **EXERCISE.** Developing My *New Ways of Being* Maintenance Plan

The form on pages 248–249 provides a format for you to develop your personal blueprint for change, My *New Ways of Being* Maintenance Plan. It might be helpful to look back at some of the exercises you have done in the workbook to remind yourself of where you began and where you find yourself now. You might like to photocopy the completed form and put it somewhere prominent so that you can remind yourself of the progress you have made and of your plans to keep yourself on track for the future.

MY *NEW WAYS OF BEING* MAINTENANCE PLAN

What have I learned through SP/SR about the development and maintenance of my problem areas and about my areas of strength?

What strategies and techniques have I learned that have helped me to develop and change?

How will I continue to strengthen my *New Ways of Being* in the future? (What techniques? Which cues and reminders?)

What internal (thoughts and emotions) or external (situational) factors might get in the way of me practicing my *New Ways of Being*?

What might lead to a setback for me and pull me back into my *Old Ways of Being* (e.g., future stresses, work problems, personal vulnerabilities, relationships, life problems)?

What early cues might alert me to this?

What will I do if I have a setback? If I see early signs of a setback, what changes might I make? How might I remind myself to use my strengths and my new corrective strategies to address potential problems?

How can I carry forward what I have learned through completing the workbook? What are my goals around future reflective practice?

What steps can I take to make reflection a regular part of my professional life? Looking back to the section in Chapter 3, "Building Your Reflective Capacity," are there some tips that may be useful?

What difficulties and challenges might I face in realizing these new goals? How will I overcome these difficulties?

Self-Reflective Questions

Which of the *New Ways of Being* strategies have been most effective in building your belief in your new ways of thinking, and creating new behaviors and underlying patterns?

_____

_____

_____

_____

_____

_____

_____

_____

_____

_____

_____

From your experience of *CBT from the Inside Out,* how do you understand the relationship between experiential and cognitive strategies, and their relative effectiveness? How do you think experiential and cognitive strategies can be best interweaved?

_____

_____

_____

_____

_____

_____

_____

_____

_____

_____

_____

_____

_____

What did you notice about creating an explicit, written My *New Ways of Being* Maintenance Plan? Were there any thoughts, emotions, or behaviors that surprised you?

_____

_____

_____

_____

_____

_____

_____

_____

_____

_____

_____

_____

_____

_____

How has developing a personal My *New Ways of Being* Maintenance Plan for yourself influenced what you might do in your therapy practice in the future?

_____

_____

_____

_____

_____

_____

_____

_____

_____

_____

_____

_____

How would you sum up your experience of *Experiencing CBT from the Inside Out*?

_____

_____

_____

_____

_____

_____

_____

_____

_____

_____

_____

_____

_____

After completing this workbook what do you consider the most important "take-home" messages to be:

From a professional perspective?

_____

_____

_____

_____

_____

_____

_____

_____

_____

_____

_____

From a personal perspective?

_____

_____

_____

_____

_____

Do you consider that it would be of value to continue with SP/SR in the future? If so, how might you do so? What steps could you take to ensure that this becomes a regular part of your professional life? Is there anything that might get in the way of this?

Module Notes

The aim of the Module Notes is to enhance the value of the workbook by providing comments and references that may deepen your understanding of CBT principles and practices. The exercises in *Experiencing CBT from the Inside Out* mostly assume that practitioners using the workbook are already acquainted with the principles and practices of CBT. However, this may not always be the case. Some practitioners will be using the workbook as part of their learning experience, while others may be well acquainted with CBT practices but want a more detailed analysis of their use.

We begin by providing six recommended core texts. These provide a strong grounding in CBT and are useful reference books to review many of the key strategies. We also recommend three advanced texts for more experienced CBT practitioners. These textbooks assume that practitioners are already competent in basic CBT techniques.

After the recommended texts are the notes for each of the 12 modules. The notes have various purposes: they expand on the rationale for the techniques featured in the module; they provide more theoretical background and further information about the interventions and their use with clients; and they direct the reader to chapters in the recommended texts and to other references that may prove useful.

Recommended Core CBT Texts

Beck, J. S. (2011). *Cognitive behavior therapy: Basics and beyond* (2nd ed.). New York: Guilford Press.

Greenberger, D., & Padesky, C. (1995). *Mind over mood: Change how you feel by changing the way you think*. New York: Guilford Press.

Kuyken, W., Padesky, C. A., & Dudley, R. (2009). *Collaborative case conceptualization: Working effectively with clients in cognitive-behavioral therapy*. New York: Guilford Press.

Persons, J. B. (2008). *The case formulation approach to cognitive-behavior therapy.* New York: Guilford Press.

Sanders, D., & Wills, F. (2005). *Cognitive therapy: An introduction.* London: Sage.

Westbrook, D., Kennerley, H., & Kirk, J. (2011). *An introduction to cognitive behaviour therapy: Skills and applications* (2nd ed.). London: Sage.

Recommended Advanced CBT Texts

Butler, G., Fennell, M., & Hackmann, A. (2008). *Cognitive-behavioral therapy for anxiety disorders: Mastering clinical challenges.* New York: Guilford Press.

Newman, C. F. (2013). *Core competencies in cognitive-behavioral therapy.* New York: Routledge.

Whittington, A., & Grey, N. (2014). *How to become a more effective therapist: Mastering metacompetence in clinical practice.* Chichester, UK: Wiley.

Module 1: Identifying a Challenging Problem

Use of Measures

CBT has always emphasized the use of measurement as a way to evaluate its effectiveness. Measurement has been used in various ways, for example, as an aid to assessment; to establish baselines; to provide feedback within treatment; and to collect objective evidence on treatment outcomes. Westbrook et al. (2011, Ch. 5) is recommended for a fuller discussion of the use of measurement within CBT.

In this module we have included the PHQ-9 (Kroenke, Spitzer, & Williams, 2001) as a basic measure for depression and the GAD-7 (Spitzer, Kroenke, Williams, & Löwe, 2006) as a proxy for a range of anxiety disorders. These are brief, freely available measures, which are widely used (e.g., as recommended measures in the English National Health Service). They may or may not be relevant to your "challenging problem." Therefore we encourage you, in addition, to source and utilize measures that are specific to your own problem area (e.g., anger, intolerance of uncertainty, lack of self-compassion) so that you are best able to evaluate the impact of your self-practice. For example, SP/SR participants in the past have utilized measures of anger (e.g., Reynolds, Walkey, & Green, 1994), intolerance of uncertainty (e.g., Buhr & Dugas, 2002) and self-compassion (e.g., Neff, 2003).

Assessment and Problem Identification

Most CBT introductory texts include a chapter describing the importance of clearly identifying and prioritizing problems that can be addressed in therapy. Problem identification is the bedrock of functional analysis, which in turn informs CBT formulations. Persons (2008), in her comprehensive book on case formulation (see "Recommended Core Texts"), emphasizes and explains the importance of the problem list as the basis for the initial case formulation. Westbrook et al. (2011, Ch. 4) also provide a detailed account of the process for describing and understanding current problems, and how these underpin assessment and formulation.

Rating Emotions Using Visual Analogue Scale

For a clear account of the use of Visual Analogue Scales see Greenberger and Padesky (1995, pp. 26–32). Beck (2011, pp. 158–166) provides further technical details for identifying emotions, distinguishing between emotions, and rating the intensity of emotions.

Further Reading

Buhr, K., & Dugas, M. J. (2002). The intolerance of uncertainty scale: Psychometric properties of the English version. *Behaviour Research and Therapy, 40*, 931–945.

Kroenke, K., Spitzer, R. L., & Williams, J. B. W. (2001). The PHQ-9: Validity of a brief depression severity measure. *Journal of General Internal Medicine, 16*, 606–613.

Neff, K. D. (2003). The development and validation of a scale to measure self-compassion. *Self and Identity, 2*, 223–250.

Reynolds, N. S., Walkey, F. H., & Green, D. E. (1994). The anger self report: A psychometrically sound (30 item) version. *New Zealand Journal of Psychology, 23*, 64–70.

Spitzer, R. L., Kroenke, K., Williams, J. B., & Löwe, B. (2006). A brief measure for assessing generalized anxiety disorder: The GAD-7. *Archives of Internal Medicine, 166*, 1092–1097.

Module 2: Formulating the Problem and Preparing for Change

The Five-Part Model

Greenberger and Padesky provide a clear account of this model, with Chapter 1 being particularly helpful. Padesky and Mooney (1990) describe the use of the model with clients. In publications subsequently, the model has been given various names, including the five-areas model, the five-factors model, and the five-systems model. If you are interested in how this model has been adapted in low intervention CBT approaches, Williams (2009) provides a good overview in *"Overcoming depression: A five areas approach."*

Understanding the Role of Culture

In the past few years, a number of CBT authors have emphasized the role of culture in helping clients and therapists to make sense of their experience, and to adapt CBT techniques for use within different cultural contexts. Hays has been a strong proponent for the integration of multicultural therapy approaches into CBT, as illustrated in Chapter 2. Her book, *Connecting Across Cultures: The Helper's Toolkit* (2013), provides details of the ADDRESSING tool and illustrates various ways of incorporating culture into everyday CBT practice. Chapter 4 in Kuyken, Padesky, and Dudley (2009) also demonstrates ways in which a client's culture can be usefully integrated into a strengths-based case conceptualization.

Using Problem Statements to Develop Formulations

The idea of a "problem statement" may be unfamiliar to some readers. The aim is to use the client's words to describe the problem, its context, and the impact that the problem is having on his or her life, in order to arrive at a shared understanding. Developed collaboratively, it becomes a useful shorthand way to capture and describe the maintenance formulation. The problem statement has been routinely utilized in low intensity CBT services in England, and now more globally. For further information, see Richards and Whyte (2011, pp. 14–15).

Including Strengths in Formulations

We have introduced a strengths-based component in the initial CBT formulation. As mentioned in Chapter 2, incorporating strengths in order to build resilience is one of the defining principles underpinning our approach to SP/SR. The idea that incorporating strengths into the case formulation is an important step toward building client resilience is elaborated in Chapter 4 of Kuyken, Padesky, and Dudley, and in Padesky and Mooney (2012).

Using Imagery to Identify Goals

Imagery can be a useful aid to effective goal setting. For a comprehensive account of the use of imagery in CBT, see Hackmann et al.'s (2011) *Oxford Guide to Imagery in Cognitive Therapy*. Pages 169–178 provide specific details on the use of imagery to create goals.

Setting SMART Goals

For further information regarding the importance of goal setting using SMART principles, see Westbrook et al. (2011, pp. 235–238).

Further Reading

Hackmann, A., Bennett-Levy, J., & Holmes, E. (2011). *Oxford guide to imagery in cognitive therapy*. Oxford, UK: Oxford University Press.

Hays, P. A. (2013). *Connecting across cultures: The helper's toolkit*. Los Angeles: Sage.

Hays, P. A., & Iwamasa, G. Y. (Eds.). (2006). *Culturally responsive cognitive-behavioral therapy: Assessment, practice, and supervision*. Washington, DC: American Psychological Association.

Padesky, C. A., & Mooney, K. A. (1990). Clinical tip: Presenting the cognitive model to clients. *International Cognitive Therapy Newsletter, 6*, 13–14. Available at *http://padesky.com/clinical-corner/publications*; click on "Fundamentals."

Padesky, C. A., & Mooney, K. A. (2012). Strengths-based cognitive–behavioural therapy: A four-step model to build resilience. *Clinical Psychology and Psychotherapy, 19*, 283–290.

Richards, D., & Whyte, M. (2011). *Reach out: National programme student materials to support the delivery of training for Psychological Wellbeing Practitioners delivering low intensity interventions* (3rd ed.). London: Rethink.

Williams, C. (2009). *Overcoming depression: A five areas approach*. London: Hodder Arnold.

Module 3: Using Behavioral Activation to Change Patterns of Behavior

Behavioral activation strategies have been a key part of CBT since Beck developed his original model of cognitive therapy for depression (Beck, Rush, Shaw, & Emery, 1979). Classical Beckian cognitive therapy includes activity scheduling early in therapy, especially for more severely depressed clients. Basic activation initially aims to break the vicious cycle of activity reduction that has led to decreased engagement with pleasurable activities and to lower mood. It does this by encouraging the monitoring of behavior and mood, exploring patterns (e.g., relationships between activity and emotions), and then scheduling meaningful activities that are likely to improve mood. As the client becomes more active, CBT therapists often use this as an opportunity to integrate behavioral experiments into the process, for example, testing out the client's beliefs about how much he or she will be able to achieve or how much enjoyment the activities may bring. They may also use ratings of pleasure and achievement to help the client identify even minor benefits gained from engaging with various activities.

More recently, behavioral activation (BA) has been developed as an evidence-based standalone intervention in its own right with a different underlying theoretical rationale based more closely on original behavioral principles. The initial activation exercises within this module are consistent with both the early use of activity scheduling in CBT and the early stages of formal BA.

Most current CBT textbooks include sections on activity scheduling or behavioral activation as one component of a wider CBT approach (e.g., Westbrook et al., 2011, pp. 254–261). Chapter 10 in *Mind over Mood* (Greenberger & Padesky, 1995) introduces the use of the Activity Schedule for clients in a manner consistent with classical CBT and also includes useful client handouts.

If you are interested in BA as a distinct approach, see Martell, Addis, and Jacobson's (2001) seminal text *Depression in Context: Strategies for Guided Action* and Martell et al.'s (2010) *Behavioral Activation for Depression: A Clinician's Guide*. There is also an excellent self-help workbook entitled *Overcoming Depression One Step at a Time* (Addis & Martell, 2004) that can be used with clients or can be completed by therapists if they would like an in-depth experience of BA.

Further Reading

Addis, M. E., & Martell, C. R. (2004). *Overcoming depression one step at a time*. Oakland, CA.: New Harbinger.

Beck, A. T., Rush, A. J., Shaw, B. F., & Emery, G. (1979). *Cognitive therapy of depression*. New York: Guilford Press.

Martell, C. R., Addis, M. E., & Jacobson, N. S. (2001). *Depression in context: Strategies for guided action*. New York: Norton.

Martell, C., Dimidjian, S., & Herman-Dunn, R. (2010). *Behavioral activation for depression: A clinician's guide*. New York: Guilford Press.

Module 4: Identifying Unhelpful Thinking and Behavior

All good CBT introductory textbooks focus on identifying cognitions and patterns of thinking and cover the five-part model. See any of the key recommended texts.

The "Downward-Arrow" Technique

The "downward-arrow" technique is well described in Greenberger and Padesky (1995, pp. 131–135) and Westbrook et al. (2011, pp. 147–149).

Using Thought Records to Identify and Record NATs

Good descriptions of the use of thought records to identify and record automatic thoughts can be found in Chapter 5 of Greenberger and Padesky (1995) and Chapter 9 of Beck (2011).

Unhelpful Patterns and Processes of Thought and Behavior

Frank and Davidson's (2014) book *The Transdiagnostic Road Map to Case Formulation and Planning* provides an excellent account of transdiagnostic processes and mechanisms, and illustrates their role in case formulation. A useful list of common cognitive biases can be found in Westbrook et al. (2011, pp. 172–174). For two interesting papers about safety behaviors, see Thwaites and Freeston (2005) on the distinction between safety behaviors and adaptive coping strategies, and Rachman, Radomsky, and Shafran (2008) on the distinction between unadaptive and judicious use of safety behaviors.

Maintenance Cycles

See Chapter 4 in Westbrook et al. (2011) for excellent examples of maintenance cycles, mapped out in diagrammatic form (e.g., safety behaviors, escape/avoidance, reduction of activity, catastrophic misinterpretation, and hypervigilance).

Further Reading

Frank, R. I., & Davidson, J. (2014). *The transdiagnostic road map to case formulation and planning: Practical guidance for clinical decision making.* Oakland, CA: New Harbinger.

Rachman, S., Radomsky, A. S., & Shafran, R. (2008). Safety behaviour: A reconsideration. *Behaviour Research and Therapy, 46*, 163–173.

Thwaites, R., & Freeston, M. (2005). Safety seeking behaviours: Fact or fiction? How can we clinically differentiate between safety behaviours and adaptive coping strategies across anxiety disorders? *Behavioural and Cognitive Psychotherapy, 33*, 1–12.

Module 5: Using Cognitive Techniques to Modify Unhelpful Thinking and Behavior

Identifying and modifying unhelpful thinking and patterns of thought and behavior lies at the very heart of CBT. The recommended key texts fully cover this topic. The focus of Module 5 is on cognitive methods of change. Experiential methods of change are featured in Modules 3 (behavioral activation), 8, 10, and 11 (behavioral experiments and other experiential methods).

Socratic Questioning

In a much-quoted conference presentation, Padesky (1993) termed Socratic questioning the "cornerstone" of CBT. Useful chapters that give good examples of different types of Socratic questions can be found in Greenberger and Padesky (1995, Ch. 6), Beck (2011, Ch. 11), and Westbrook et al. (2011, Ch. 7).

Expanded Formulation

The expanded formulation diagram is an adaptation of a formulation diagram in Westbook et al. (2011, Ch.4). Comprehensive accounts of ways to construct formulations can be found in Persons (2008) and Kuyken et al. (2009)—see "Recommended Core CBT Texts."

Sanders and Wills (2005) provide useful accounts of working with cognitive content and processes.

Further Reading

Padesky, C. A. (1993, September). *Socratic questioning: Changing minds or guided discovery?* Paper presented at the European Congress of Behavioural and Cognitive Therapies, London. Available at *http://padesky.com/clinical-corner/publications*; click on "Fundamentals."

Module 6: Reviewing Progress

Module 6 reviews goals and the Visual Analogue Scale, as described in Modules 1 and 2, before addressing roadblocks to doing SP/SR and problem-solving strategies.

Roadblocks to Doing SP/SR

We adapted the Beck, Rush, Shaw, and Emery (1979, p. 408) Possible Reasons for Not Doing Self-Help Assignments Questionnaire to enable participants to recognize that there might be a number of issues that could get in the way of doing SP/SR homework. Other kinds of resistance that might interfere with progress, particularly those related to interpersonal issues, are addressed in Leahy's (2001) *Overcoming Resistance in Cognitive Therapy*. Beck (2011, Ch. 17) has a helpful discussion about homework with ideas for increasing "homework adherence." For a fuller account of the use of homework in CBT, see Kazantzis, Deane, Ronan, and L'Abate (2005).

Problem Solving

Brief introductions to structured problem solving can be found in Westbrook et al. (2011, pp. 264–266) and Sanders and Wills (2005, pp. 131–132). For a more detailed description of the process, see Nezu, Nezu, and D'Zurilla (2012).

Further Reading

Beck, A. T., Rush, J. A., Shaw, B. F., & Emery, G. (1979). *Cognitive therapy for depression.* New York: Guilford Press.

Kazantzis, N., Deane, F. P., Ronan, K. R., & L'Abate, L. (2005). *Using homework assignments in cognitive behavior therapy.* New York: Routledge.

Leahy, R. L. (2001). *Overcoming resistance in cognitive therapy.* New York: Guilford Press.

Nezu, A. M., Nezu, C. M., & D'Zurilla, T. J. (2012). *Problem-solving therapy: A treatment manual.* New York: Springer.

Module 7: Identifying Unhelpful Assumptions and Constructing New Alternatives

Levels of Thought

Most introductory CBT texts identify three levels of thought: automatic thoughts, underlying assumptions (sometimes referred to as intermediate beliefs), and core beliefs; for example, see Beck (2011, Ch. 3) and Greenberger and Padesky (1995, Ch. 9).

Underlying Assumptions

Identifying underlying assumptions and "rules for living" and shaping them into explicit statements is an important CBT skill. Assumptions and rules often provide the basis for behavioral experiments (see Modules 8 and 11). Sanders and Wills (2005, pp. 137–143) and Beck (2011, Ch. 13) provide helpful overviews of the role of underlying assumptions in CBT and suggest ways to identify them (Beck terms these "intermediate beliefs"). For a specific description of the role of underlying assumptions in the treatment of anxiety disorders, see Butler, Fennell, and Hackmann (2008, Ch. 2).

Module 8: Using Behavioral Experiments to Test Unhelpful Assumptions against New Alternatives

Behavioral Experiments

Most SP/SR participants will be well acquainted with exposure as an important intervention in CBT. However, some may not be quite so well acquainted with behavioral experiments. We suggest that they should be! Research studies indicate that behavioral experiments are one of the most powerful interventions in CBT (Bennett-Levy et al., 2004). They appear to be more effective than automatic thought records (Bennett-Levy, 2003; McManus, Van Doorn, & Yiend, 2012), and more effective than exposure in certain contexts, particularly with clients with social anxiety (Clark et al., 2006; McMillan & Lee, 2010; Ougrin, 2011).

There are important differences between exposure and behavioral experiments. Exposure is based in a behavioral paradigm. The client is exposed to a feared stimulus, and contact is maintained until the fear habituates. Behavioral experiments are based in a cognitive-behavioral paradigm. They are designed to test thoughts, assumptions, or beliefs about self, others, or the world through planned experiential activities. Put simply, the exposure paradigm would suggest that the person who is phobic of public speaking should engage with public speaking opportunities until his or her fear habituates. The behavioral experiments paradigm suggests that exposure alone may not be sufficient; the fear will not habituate *unless the beliefs sustaining the phobia are successfully identified, challenged, or disconfirme*d (e.g., "If I give a talk, people will see how stupid I am" or "I'll turn bright red and look like a complete idiot" or "I'll lose my train of thought and end up just standing there like a statue"). Behavioral experiments therefore target and test the individual's idiosyncratic beliefs.

Another key difference between exposure and behavioral experiments is that the exposure paradigm is largely limited to the treatment of anxiety disorders, whereas behavioral experiments can be established to test the beliefs of any client with any disorder (e.g., "If I get out of bed, I'll only get more depressed"). In other words, behavioral experiments are more versatile and wide-ranging interventions than exposure.

A key reference to the theory, design, and practice of behavioral experiments is Bennett-Levy et al.'s (2004) *Oxford Guide to Behavioural Experiments in Cognitive Therapy*. Useful summary chapters may also be found in Westbrook et al. (2011, Ch. 9) and Butler et al. (2008, Ch. 6).

The "Head" versus "Heart" or "Gut" Distinction

All CBT therapists will be familiar with clients who say: "I know this intellectually but . . . in my heart . . . my gut reaction is. . . ." As we indicated in Chapter 2, there are good theoretical grounds for suggesting that the dissociation between "head" and "heart" or "gut"-level beliefs is a function of different modes and levels of information processing. Teasdale and Barnard's Interacting Cognitive Subsystem's (ICS) model—see Chapter 2 and the Teasdale and Barnard references at the end of the book—suggests that experiential techniques such as behavioral experiments, imagery, and body-oriented interventions are likely to be more successful at creating "gut-level" change than more rationalistic cognitive techniques without an experiential component. Stott (2007) provides an interesting discussion of "head" and "heart" differences and their implication for CBT.

In Module 8 and several other modules, we highlight the differences between "head"- and "heart"- or "gut"-level beliefs by asking participants to make separate ratings, so that participants can experience these differences for themselves and reflect on the implications for treatment. It is too early to say whether there are meaningful differences between different "body beliefs" (e.g., "gut" vs. "heart"), but some research suggests that there may be (Nummenmaa et al., 2014), with "gut-level" beliefs being particularly associated with the emotions of fear, anxiety, and disgust.

Further Reading

Bennett-Levy, J. (2003). Mechanisms of change in cognitive therapy: The case of automatic thought records and behavioural experiments. *Behavioural and Cognitive Psychotherapy, 31,* 261–277.

Bennett-Levy, J., Butler, G., Fennell, M., Hackmann, A., Mueller, M., & Westbrook, D. (Eds.). (2004). *The Oxford guide to behavioural experiments in cognitive therapy.* Oxford, UK: Oxford University Press.

Clark, D. M., Ehlers, A., Hackmann, A., McManus, F., Fennell, M., Grey, N., et al. (2006). Cognitive therapy versus exposure and applied relaxation in social phobia: A randomized controlled trial. *Journal of Consulting and Clinical Psychology, 74,* 568–578.

McManus, F., Van Doorn, K., & Yiend, J. (2012). Examining the effects of thought records and behavioral experiments in instigating belief change. *Journal of Behavior Therapy and Experimental Psychiatry, 43,* 540–547.

McMillan, D., & Lee, R. (2010). A systematic review of behavioral experiments vs. exposure alone in the treatment of anxiety disorders: A case of exposure while wearing the emperor's new clothes? *Clinical Psychology Review, 30,* 467–478.

Nummenmaa, L., Glerean, E., Hari, R., & Hietanend, J. K. (2014). Bodily map of emotions. *Proceedings of the National Academy of Sciences, 111,* 646–651.

Ougrin, D. (2011). Efficacy of exposure versus cognitive therapy in anxiety disorders: Systematic review and meta-analysis. *BMC Psychiatry, 11,* 200.

Stott, R. (2007). When head and heart do not agree: A theoretical and clinical analysis of rational-emotional dissociation (RED) in cognitive therapy. *Journal of Cognitive Psychotherapy: An International Quarterly, 21,* 37–50.

Module 9: Constructing *New Ways of Being*

The *Ways of Being* Model: *Old* and *New Ways of Being*

The *Ways of Being* model has been developed during the writing of *Experiencing CBT from the Inside Out.* The first time one of us used the term *New Ways of Being* in a publication was in Hackmann, Bennett-Levy, and Holmes (2011). We have expanded on the ideas in Hackmann et al. to embrace a schema-based approach, grounded in Teasdale and Barnard's ICS model. The theoretical and clinical rationale for the *Ways of Being* model is described in Chapter 2. In particular, we acknowledge the influence on our thinking of Teasdale and Barnard, Brewin, Padesky and Mooney, and Korrelboom.

One of our realizations in developing the *Ways of Being* model has been that the term "schema" has mostly been interpreted by CBT therapists as referring to negatives: negative core beliefs and/or negative associated emotions and behaviors (see James, Goodman, & Reichelt, 2014, for further discussion). However, it is quite apparent that human beings have both helpful and unhelpful schemas; and that many of these schemas are not necessarily at a core-belief level. They are ways of doing things and rules that we have picked up through practice and experience. Experienced therapists have many automatized, largely unconscious schemas, which they "wheel in" and "wheel out" when they see clients with different presentations. Their thinking is accompanied by a set of behaviors, emotions, and bodily reactions, which are consistent and predictable across similar situations. When certain of these schema are not as functional or effective as others, they might become a "challenging problem" of the type that therapists might address in SP/SR. Do these schema require attention? Probably. Do they require attention at a "core-belief" level? In many cases, probably not.

The Disk Model Representation of *Old* and *New Ways of Being*

We wanted to represent the *Ways of Being* model in a holistic way. After some experimentation, we opted for a "concentric circles" approach rather than what is sometimes termed the "central heating diagram" (!) format of more typical CBT formulations. This is consistent with Teasdale and Barnard's ICS model, which implies that schemas are "wheeled in" and "wheeled out" as a package of cognitions, emotions, bodily sensations, and behaviors. It therefore seemed appropriate to represent these elements both as close neighbors *and* as part of a coherent whole. A disk of dotted concentric circles appeared to be the way to do this. The disk may also be more memorable for clients than our usual formulation diagrams.

In the representation of the *New Ways of Being*, we have introduced Personal Strengths into the center of the diagram since strengths are at the core of the *New Ways of Being*. See also the Chapter 2 discussion of the disk model.

The *New Ways of Being* Record Book

Initially, we envisaged using the Positive Data Log (Greenberger & Padesky, 1995, pp. 143–144) to record evidence of the *New Ways of Being*. However, we soon realized that the notion of *New Ways of Being* extended way beyond collecting evidence for a new set of beliefs. Being schema-based, the *New Ways of Being* encompass new behaviors, new cognitions, new underlying patterns, and new ways of engaging with body and emotions. Accordingly, the *New Ways of Being* Record Book is used to record process as well as outcomes—new ways of doing things are important in themselves, regardless of whether they have any measurable effect on beliefs.

Further Reading

Hackmann, A., Bennett-Levy, J., & Holmes, E. A. (2011). *The Oxford guide to imagery in cognitive therapy.* Oxford, UK: Oxford University Press.

James, I. A., Goodman, M., & Reichelt, F. K. (2014). What clinicians can learn from schema change in sport. *The Cognitive Behaviour Therapist, 6*, e14.

Teasdale, J. D. (1996). Clinically relevant theory: Integrating clinical insight with cognitive science. In P. M. Salkovskis (Ed.), *Frontiers of cognitive therapy* (pp. 26–47). New York: Guilford Press.

Teasdale, J. D. (1999). Emotional processing, three modes of mind and the prevention of relapse in depression. *Behaviour Research and Therapy, 37*, S53–S77.

Module 10: Embodying *New Ways of Being*

This module features the work of Korrelboom and colleagues' Competitive Memory Training (COMET). Chapter 2 describes the rationale for COMET, and its links to Brewin's retrieval competition account of memory availability. Korrelboom's work encompasses narrative, imagery, body movement, and music. It offers the kind of experiential approach that Teasdale suggests should impact at a "heart" or "gut" level if practiced on a regular basis. The value of the COMET approach is also suggested by research demonstrating a positive impact on mood from memories of past successes (Biondolillo & Pillemer, in press), positive imagery (Pictet,

Coughtrey, Mathews, & Holmes, 2011), body movement (Michalak, Mischnat, & Teismann, in press) and music (Sarkamo, Tervaniemi, Laitinen et al., 2008).

Further Reading

Biondolillo, M. J., & Pillemer, D. B. (in press). Using memories to motivate future behaviour: An experimental exercise intervention. *Memory.*

Korrelboom, K., Maarsingh, M., & Huijbrechts, I. (2012). Competitive memory training (COMET) for treating low self-esteem in patients with depressive disorders: A randomized clinical trial. *Depression and Anxiety, 29,* 102–112.

Korrelboom, K., Marissen, M., & van Assendelft, T. (2011). Competitive memory training (COMET) for low self-esteem in patients with personality disorders: A randomized effectiveness study. *Behavioural and Cognitive Psychotherapy, 39,* 1–19.

Michalak, J., Mischnat, J., & Teismann, T. (in press). Sitting posture makes a difference—Embodiment effects on depressive memory bias. *Clinical Psychology and Psychotherapy.*

Pictet, A., Coughtrey, A. E., Mathews, A., & Holmes, E. A. (2011). Fishing for happiness: The effects of generating positive imagery on mood and behaviour. *Behaviour Research and Therapy, 49,* 885–891.

Sarkamo, T., Tervaniemi, M., Laitinen, S., Forsblom, A., Soinila, S., Mikkonen, M., et al. (2008). Music listening enhances cognitive recovery and mood after middle cerebral artery stroke. *Brain, 131,* 866–876.

Module 11: Using Behavioral Experiments
to Test and Strengthen *New Ways of Being*

Behavioral Experiments to Test *New Ways of Being*

There are three ways to set up hypothesis-testing behavioral experiments. We can either test the old assumption (Hypothesis A), or compare an old assumption with a new assumption (Hypothesis A vs. Hypothesis B), as in Module 8. Or we can simply set out to build evidence for a new assumption (Hypothesis B). This last option is the focus of Module 11.

As noted in Chapter 2, it is not simply enough to test a new assumption. Teasdale and Barnard's ICS model suggests that the mind-set through which we process the impact of experiential strategies is crucial. If we process an experience through an *Old Ways of Being* mind-set (e.g., "I felt nervous during my talk but got away with it"), we are left in a rather different position from processing the experience through a *New Ways of Being* mind-set (e.g., "I felt nervous during my talk, but controlled my nerves, and people seemed really receptive to what I had to say"). A *New Ways of Being* perspective tends to open the mind to different kinds of information that would otherwise be discounted or ignored by an *Old Ways* frame of reference. Hence the importance of behavioral experiments focused purely on building evidence for Hypothesis B. The mind-set through which the experience is processed determines the information that gets processed.

Creating a Summary Image, Metaphor, or Drawing

The inclusion of the summary image, metaphor, icon, and/or drawing in Module 11 is largely due to the work of Padesky and Mooney (2000, 2012) who have consistently emphasized the value of images and metaphors as a summary or reminder in their Old System/New System model. Gilbert's (2005, 2013) compassionate mind training has also emphasized the value of imagery in creating a more compassionate self. See Hackmann et al. (2011, Ch. 13) for examples of the use of imagery to create and build *New Ways of Being*, drawn from the work of Padesky and Mooney, Gilbert, and Korrelboom. For further information about the use of metaphor in CBT, see Stott, Mansell, Salkovskis, Lavender, and Cartwright-Hatton (2010). Drawing, painting, and other art forms also provide a medium to encapsulate meanings at a symbolic level. This approach is well articulated in a chapter by Butler and Holmes (2009).

Further Reading

Butler, G., & Holmes, E. A. (2009). Imagery and the self following childhood trauma: Observations concerning the use of drawings and external images. In L. Stopa (Ed.), *Imagery and the damaged self: Perspectives on imagery in cognitive therapy* (pp. 166–180). New York: Routledge.

Gilbert, P. (Ed.). (2005). *Compassion: Conceptualisations, research and use in psychotherapy.* Hove, UK: Routledge.

Gilbert, P., & Choden. (2013). *Mindful compassion.* London: Robinson.

Hackmann, A., Bennett-Levy, J., & Holmes, E. A. (2011). *The Oxford guide to imagery in cognitive therapy.* Oxford, UK: Oxford University Press.

Mooney, K. A., & Padesky, C. A. (2000). Applying client creativity to recurrent problems: Constructing possibilities and tolerating doubt. *Journal of Cognitive Psychotherapy, 14,* 149–161.

Padesky, C. A., & Mooney, K. A. (2012). Strengths-based cognitive–behavioural therapy: A four-step model to build resilience. *Clinical Psychology and Psychotherapy, 19,* 283–290.

Stott, R., Mansell, W., Salkovskis, P., Lavender, A., & Cartwright-Hatton, S. (2010). *Oxford guide to metaphors in CBT: Building cognitive bridges.* Oxford, UK: Oxford University Press.

Module 12: Maintaining and Enhancing *New Ways of Being*

Relapse Prevention/Maintaining and Enhancing *New Ways of Being*

Relapse prevention is a key element in the delivery of successful CBT. Relapse-prevention strategies are founded on the idea that the client has it within him- or herself to become his or her own therapist. See Sanders and Wills (2005, Ch. 9), Beck (2011, Ch. 18), and Newman (2013, Ch. 9) for useful tips about ending treatment and relapse prevention.

From a *New Ways of Being* perspective, the purpose of the final module(s) is more to maintain and enhance *New Ways of Being* than to prevent relapse. However, the basic strategy of reviewing learning and considering implications for the future remains broadly the same.

The *New Ways of Being* Maintenance Plan

The *New Ways of Being* Maintenance Plan closely follows the kind of "blueprint" plans that CBT therapists often use in the final session(s) of therapy. Written plans to prevent relapse in the event of challenges or difficulties, or to maintain and enhance *New Ways of Being*, serve as a positive reminder of what to do to keep the momentum going. Butler et al. (2008, Ch. 10) provide a particularly helpful and detailed description of the use of blueprints in the context of clients with anxiety disorders. Sanders and Wills (2005, p. 190) also give an example of a simple blueprint form.

References

1. Padesky, C. A. (1996). Developing cognitive therapist competency: Teaching and supervision models. In P. M. Salkovskis (Ed.), *Frontiers of cognitive therapy* (pp. 266–292). New York: Guilford Press.

2. Bennett-Levy, J., & Lee, N. (2014). Self-practice and self-reflection in cognitive behaviour therapy training: What factors influence trainees' engagement and experience of benefit? *Behavioural and Cognitive Psychotherapy, 42,* 48–64.

3. Bennett-Levy, J., Turner, F., Beaty, T., Smith, M., Paterson, B., & Farmer, S. (2001). The value of self-practice of cognitive therapy techniques and self-reflection in the training of cognitive therapists. *Behavioural and Cognitive Psychotherapy, 29,* 203–220.

4. Beck, A. T., & Freeman, A., & Associates. (1990). *Cognitive therapy of personality disorders.* New York: Guilford Press.

5. Beck, J. S. (1995). *Cognitive therapy: Basics and beyond.* New York: Guilford Press.

6. Friedberg, R. D., & Fidaleo, R. A. (1992). Training inpatient staff in cognitive therapy. *Journal of Cognitive Psychotherapy, 6,* 105–112.

7. Wills, F., & Sanders, D. (1997). *Cognitive therapy: Transforming the image.* London: Sage.

8. Safran, J. D., & Segal, Z. V. (1990). *Interpersonal processes in cognitive therapy.* New York: Basic Books.

9. Sanders, D., & Bennett-Levy, J. (2010). When therapists have problems: What can CBT do for us? In M. Mueller, H. Kennerley, F. McManus, & D. Westbrook (Eds.), *The Oxford guide to surviving as a CBT therapist* (pp. 457–480). Oxford, UK: Oxford University Press.

10. Beck, J. S. (2011). *Cognitive behavior therapy: Basics and beyond* (2nd ed.). New York: Guilford Press.

11. Kuyken, W., Padesky, C. A., & Dudley, R. (2009). *Collaborative case conceptualization: Working effectively with clients in cognitive-behavioral therapy.* New York: Guilford Press.

12. Newman, C. F. (2013). *Core competencies in cognitive-behavioral therapy.* New York: Routledge.

13. Bennett-Levy, J., Lee, N., Travers, K., Pohlman, S., & Hamernik, E. (2003). Cognitive therapy from the inside: Enhancing therapist skills through practising what we preach. *Behavioural and Cognitive Psychotherapy, 31,* 145–163.

14. Bennett-Levy, J., Thwaites, R., Chaddock, A., & Davis, M. (2009). Reflective practice in cognitive

behavioural therapy: The engine of lifelong learning. In J. Stedmon & R. Dallos (Eds.), *Reflective practice in psychotherapy and counselling. Maidenhead* (pp. 115–135). Berkshire, UK: Open University Press.

15. Davis, M., Thwaites, R., Freeston, M., & Bennett-Levy, J. (in press). A measurable impact of a self-practice/self-reflection programme on the therapeutic skills of experienced cognitive-behavioural therapists. *Clinical Psychology and Psychotherapy.*

16. Thwaites, R., Bennett-Levy, J., Davis, M., & Chaddock, A. (2014). Using self-practice and self-reflection (SP/SR) to enhance CBT competence and meta-competence. In A. Whittington, & N. Grey (Eds.), *The cognitive behavioural therapist: From theory to clinical practice* (pp. 241–254). Chichester, UK: Wiley-Blackwell.

17. Haarhoff, B., & Farrand, P. (2012). Reflective and self-evaluative practice in CBT. In W. Dryden & R. Branch (Eds.), *The CBT handbook* (pp. 475–492). London: Sage.

18. Haarhoff, B., Gibson, K., & Flett, R. (2011). Improving the quality of cognitive behaviour therapy case conceptualization: The role of self-practice/self-reflection. *Behavioural and Cognitive Psychotherapy, 39,* 323–339.

19. Farrand, P., Perry, J., & Linsley, S. (2010). Enhancing Self-Practice/Self-Reflection (SP/SR) approach to cognitive behaviour training through the use of reflective blogs. *Behavioural and Cognitive Psychotherapy, 38,* 473–477.

20. Chellingsworth, M., & Farrand, P. (2013, July). *Is level of reflective ability in SP/SR a predictor of clinical competency?* British Association of Behavioural and Cognitive Psychotherapy Conference, London.

21. Chigwedere, C., Fitzmaurice, B., & Donohue, G. (2013, September). *Can SP/SR be a credible equivalent for personal therapy? A preliminary qualitative analysis.* European Association of Behavioural and Cognitive Therapies, Marrakesh, Morocco.

22. Gale, C., & Schroder, T. (in press). Experiences of self-practice/self-reflection in cognitive behavioural therapy: A meta-synthesis of qualitative studies. *Psychology and Psychotherapy.*

23. Fraser, N., & Wilson, J. (2010). Self-case study as a catalyst for personal development in cognitive therapy training. *The Cognitive Behaviour Therapist, 3,* 107–116.

24. Fraser, N., & Wilson, J. (2011). Students' stories of challenges and gains in learning cognitive therapy. *New Zealand Journal of Counselling, 31,* 79–95.

25. Chaddock, A., Thwaites, R., Freeston, M., & Bennett-Levy, J. (in press). Understanding individual differences in response to Self-Practice and Self-Reflection (SP/SR) during CBT training. *The Cognitive Behaviour Therapist, 7,* e14.

26. Schneider, K., & Rees, C. (2012). Evaluation of a combined cognitive behavioural therapy and interpersonal process group in the psychotherapy training of clinical psychologists. *Australian Psychologist, 47,* 137–146.

27. Cartwright, C. (2011). Transference, countertransference, and reflective practice in cognitive therapy. *Clinical Psychologist, 15,* 112–120.

28. Laireiter, A.-R., & Willutzki, U. (2003). Self-reflection and self-practice in training of cognitive behaviour therapy: An overview. *Clinical Psychology and Psychotherapy, 10,* 19–30.

29. Laireiter, A.-R., & Willutzki, U. (2005). Personal therapy in cognitive-behavioural therapy: Tradition and current practice. In J. D. Geller, J. C. Norcross, D. E. Orlinsky (Eds.), *The psychotherapist's own psychotherapy: Patient and clinician perspectives* (pp. 41–51). Oxford, UK: Oxford University Press.

30. Schön, D. A. (1987). *Educating the reflective practitioner.* San Francisco: Jossey-Bass.

31. Skovholt, T. M., & Rønnestad, M. H. (2001). The long, textured path from novice to senior practitioner. In T. M. Skovholt (Ed.), *The resilient practitioner: Burnout prevention and self-care strategies for counselors, therapists, teachers, and health professionals.* Boston: Allyn & Bacon.

32. Sutton, L., Townend, M., & Wright, J. (2007). The experiences of reflective learning journals by cognitive behavioural psychotherapy students. *Reflective Practice, 8,* 387–404.

33. Milne, D. L., Leck, C., & Choudhri, N. Z. (2009). Collusion in clinical supervision: Literature review and case study in self-reflection. *The Cognitive Behaviour Therapist, 2,* 106–114.

34. Bennett-Levy, J. (2006). Therapist skills: A cognitive model of their acquisition and refinement. *Behavioural and Cognitive Psychotherapy, 34,* 57–78.

35. Bennett-Levy, J., & Thwaites, R. (2007). Self and self-reflection in the therapeutic relationship: A conceptual map and practical strategies for the training, supervision and self-supervision of interpersonal skills. In P. Gilbert & R. Leahy (Eds.), *The therapeutic relationship in the cognitive behavioural psychotherapies* (pp. 255–281). London: Routledge.

36. Niemi, P., & Tiuraniemi, J. (2010). Cognitive therapy trainees' self-reflections on their professional learning. *Behavioural and Cognitive Psychotherapy, 38,* 255 –274.

37. Bennett-Levy, J., McManus, F., Westling, B., & Fennell, M. J. V. (2009). Acquiring and refining CBT skills and competencies: Which training methods are perceived to be most effective? *Behavioural and Cognitive Psychotherapy, 37,* 571–583.

38. Kazantzis, N., Reinecke, M. A., & Freeman, A. (2010). *Cognitive and behavioral theories in clinical practice.* New York: Guilford Press.

39. Teasdale, J. D. (1996). Clinically relevant theory: Integrating clinical insight with cognitive science. In P. M. Salkovskis (Ed.), *Frontiers of cognitive therapy* (pp. 26–47). New York: Guilford Press.

40. Teasdale, J. D. (1997). The transformation of meaning: The Interacting Cognitive Subsystems approach. In M. Power & C. R. Brewin (Eds.), *Meaning in psychological therapies: Integrating theory and practice* (pp. 141–156). New York: Wiley.

41. Teasdale, J. D. (1997). The relationship between cognition and emotion: The mind-in-place in mood disorders. In D. M. Clark & C. G. Fairburn (Eds.), *The science and practice of cognitive behaviour therapy* (pp. 67–93). Oxford, UK: Oxford University Press.

42. Teasdale, J. D. (1999). Emotional processing, three modes of mind and the prevention of relapse in depression. *Behaviour Research and Therapy, 37,* S53–S77.

43. Teasdale, J. D. (1999). Multi-level theories of cognition-emotion relations. In T. Dalgleish & M. Power (Eds.), *Handbook of cognition and emotion* (pp. 665–681). New York: Wiley.

44. Teasdale, J. D, & Barnard, P. J. (1993). *Affect, cognition and change: Re-modelling depressive thought.* Hove, UK: Erlbaum.

45. Brewin, C. R. (2006). Understanding cognitive behaviour therapy: A retrieval competition account. *Behaviour Research and Therapy, 44,* 765–784.

46. Mooney, K. A., & Padesky, C. A. (2000). Applying client creativity to recurrent problems: Constructing possibilities and tolerating doubt. *Journal of Cognitive Psychotherapy, 14,* 149–161.

47. Padesky, C. A. (2005, June). *The next phase: Building positive qualities with cognitive therapy.* Paper presented at the 5th International Congress of Cognitive Psychotherapy, Gotenburg, Sweden.

48. Padesky, C. A., & Mooney, K. A. (2012). Strengths-based cognitive–behavioural therapy: A four-step model to build resilience. *Clinical Psychology and Psychotherapy, 19,* 283–290.

49. Ekkers, W., Korrelboom, K., Huijbrechts, I., Smits, N., Cuijpers, P., & van der Gaag, M. (2011). Competitive memory training for treating depression and rumination in depressed older adults: A randomized controlled trial. *Behaviour Research and Therapy, 49,* 588–596.

50. Korrelboom, K., de Jong, M., Huijbrechts, I., & Daansen, P. (2009). Competitive memory training (COMET) for treating low self-esteem in patients with eating disorders: A randomized clinical trial. *Journal of Consulting Clinical Psychology, 77,* 974–980.

51. Korrelboom, K., Maarsingh, M., & Huijbrechts, I. (2012). Competitive memory training (COMET) for treating low self-esteem in patients with depressive disorders: A randomized clinical trial. *Depression and Anxiety, 29,* 102–112.

52. Korrelboom, K., Marissen, M., & van Assendelft, T. (2011). Competitive memory training (COMET) for low self-esteem in patients with personality disorders: A randomized effectiveness study. *Behavioural and Cognitive Psychotherapy, 39,* 1–19.

53. van der Gaag, M., van Oosterhout, B., Daalman, K., Sommer, I. E., & Korrelboom, K. (2012). Initial evaluation of the effects of competitive memory training (COMET) on depression in schizophrenia-spectrum patients with persistent auditory verbal hallucinations: A randomized controlled trial. *British Journal of Clinical Psychology, 51,* 158–171.

54. Hackmann, A., Bennett-Levy, J., & Holmes, E. A. (2011). *The Oxford guide to imagery in cognitive therapy.* Oxford, UK: Oxford University Press.

55. Persons, J. B. (2008). *The case formulation approach to cognitive-behavior therapy.* New York: Guilford Press.

56. Beck, A. T. (1976). *Cognitive therapy and the emotional disorders.* New York: International Universities Press.

57. Beck, A. T., Rush, A. J., Shaw, B. F., & Emery, G. (1979). *Cognitive therapy of depression.* New York: Guilford Press.

58. Kuehlwein, K. T. (2000). Enhancing creativity in cognitive therapy. *Journal of Cognitive Psychotherapy, 14,* 175–187.

59. Beck, A. T, Emery, G., & Greenberg, R. L. (1985). *Anxiety disorders and phobias: A cognitive perspective.* New York: Basic Books.

60. Harvey, A. G., Watkins, E., Mansell, W., & Shafran, R. (2004). *Cognitive behavioural processes across psychological disorders: A transdiagnostic approach to research and treatment.* Oxford, UK: Oxford University Press.

61. Hawton, K., Salkovskis, P., Kirk, J., & Clark, D. (1989). *Cognitive behaviour therapy for psychiatric problems.* Oxford, UK: Oxford University Press.

62. Salkovskis, P. M. (Ed.). (1996). *Frontiers of cognitive therapy.* New York: Guilford Press.

63. Barlow, D. H., Allen, L. B., Choate, M. L. (2004). Toward a unified treatment for emotional disorders. *Behavior Therapy, 35,* 205–230.

64. Barlow, D. H., Farchione, T. J., Fairholme, C. P., Ellard, K. K., Boisseau, C. L., Allen, L. B., et al. (2011). *Unified protocol for transdiagnostic treatment of emotional disorders: Therapist guide.* New York: Oxford University Press.

65. Frank, R. I., & Davidson, J. (2014). *The transdiagnostic road map to case formulation and treatment planning.* Oakland, CA: New Harbinger.

66. Farchione, T. J., Fairholme, C. P., Ellard, K. K., Boisseau, C. L., Thompson-Hollands, J., Carl, J. R., et al. (2012). Unified protocol for transdiagnostic treatment of emotional disorders: A randomized controlled trial. *Behavior Therapy, 43,* 666–678.

67. Titov, N., Dear, B. F., Schwencke, G., Andrews, G., Johnston, L., Craske, M. G., et al. (2011). Transdiagnostic internet treatment for anxiety and depression: A randomised controlled trial. *Behaviour Research and Therapy, 49,* 441–452.

68. Frederickson, B. (2009). *Positivity.* New York: Crown.

69. Seligman, M. E., Steen, T. A., Park, N., & Peterson, C. (2005). Positive psychology progress: Empirical validation of interventions. *American Psychologist, 60,* 410–421.

70. Sin, N. L., & Lyubomirsky, S. (2009). Enhancing well-being and alleviating depressive symptoms with positive psychology interventions: A practice-friendly meta-analysis. *Journal of Clinical Psychology, 65,* 467–487.

71. Snyder, C. R., Lopez, S. J., & Pedrotti, J. T. (2011). *Positive psychology: The scientific and practical explorations of human strengths* (2nd ed.). Los Angeles: Sage.

72. Wood, A. M., Froh, J. J., & Geraghty, A. W. (2010). Gratitude and well-being: A review and theoretical integration. *Clinical Psychology Review, 30,* 890–905.

73. Cheavens, J. S., Strunk, D. R., Lazarus, S. A., & Goldstein, L. A. (2012). The compensation and capitalization models: A test of two approaches to individualizing the treatment of depression. *Behaviour Research and Therapy, 50,* 699–706.

74. Vilhauer, J. S., Young, S., Kealoha, C., Borrmann, J., IsHak, W. W., Rapaport, M. H., et al. (2012). Treating major depression by creating positive expectations for the future: A pilot study for the

effectiveness of future-directed therapy (FDT) on symptom severity and quality of life. *CNS Neurosciences and Therapeutics, 18*, 102–109.

75. Hays, P. A. (2012). *Connecting across cultures: The helper's toolkit.* Thousand Oaks, CA: Sage.

76. Naeem, F., & Kingdon, D. G. (Eds.). (2012). *Cognitve behaviour therapy in non-western cultures.* Hauppage, NY: Nova Science.

77. De Coteau, T., Anderson, J., & Hope, D. (2006). Adapting manualized treatments: Treating anxiety disorders among Native Americans. *Cognitive and Behavioral Practice, 13*, 304–309.

78. Grey, N., & Young, K. (2008). Cognitive behaviour therapy with refugees and asylum seekers experiencing traumatic stress symptoms. *Behavioural and Cognitive Psychotherapy, 36*, 3–19.

79. Bennett-Levy, J., Wilson, S., Nelson, J., Stirling, J., Ryan, K., Rotumah, D., et al. (2014). Can CBT be effective for Aboriginal Australians? Perspectives of Aboriginal practitioners trained in CBT. *Australian Psychologist, 49*, 1–7.

80. Naeem, F., Waheed, W., Gobbi, M., Ayub, M., & Kingdon, D. (2011). Preliminary evaluation of culturally sensitive CBT for depression in Pakistan: Findings from Developing Culturally-sensitive CBT Project (DCCP). *Behavioural and Cognitive Psychotherapy, 39*, 165–173.

81. Rathod, S., Phiri, P., Harris, S., Underwood, C., Thagadur, M., Padmanabi, U., et al. (2013). Cognitive behaviour therapy for psychosis can be adapted for minority ethnic groups: A randomised controlled trial. *Schizophrenia Research, 143*, 319–326.

82. Alatiq, Y. (2014). Transdiagnostic cognitive behavioural therapy (CBT): Case reports from Saudi Arabia. *The Cognitive Behaviour Therapist, 7*, e2.

83. Hays, P. (2009). Integrating evidence-based practice, cognitive-behavior therapy, and multicultural therapy: Ten steps for culturally competent practice. *Professional Psychology: Research and Practice, 40*, 254–360.

84. Hays, P. A., & Iwamasa, G. Y. (Eds.). (2006). *Culturally responsive cognitive-behavioral therapy: Assessment, practice, and supervision.* Washington, DC: American Psychological Association.

85. Bennett-Levy, J. (2003). Mechanisms of change in cognitive therapy: The case of automatic thought records and behavioural experiments. *Behavioural and Cognitive Psychotherapy, 31*, 261–277.

86. McManus, F., Van Doorn, K., & Yiend, J. (2012). Examining the effects of thought records and behavioral experiments in instigating belief change. *Journal of Behavior Therapy and Experimental Psychiatry, 43*, 540–547.

87. Padesky, C. A. (2005, May). *Constructing a new self: A cognitive therapy approach to personality disorders.* Workshop presented at the Institute of Education, London.

88. Korrelboom, K., van der Weele, K., Gjaltema, M., & Hoogstraten, C. (2009). Competitive memory training for treating low self-esteem: A pilot study in a routine clinical setting. *The Behavior Therapist, 32*, 3–8.

89. Bennett-Levy, J., Butler, G., Fennell, M., Hackmann, A., Mueller, M., & Westbrook, D. (Eds.). (2004). *The Oxford guide to behavioural experiments in cognitive therapy.* Oxford, UK: Oxford University Press.

90. James, I. A., Goodman, M., & Reichelt, F. K. (2014). What clinicians can learn from schema change in sport. *The Cognitive Behaviour Therapist, 6*, e14.

91. James, I. A. (2001). Schema therapy: The next generation, but should it carry a health warning? *Behavioural and Cognitive Psychotherapy, 29*, 401–407.

92. Fennell, M. (2004). Depression, low self-esteem and mindfulness. *Behaviour Research and Therapy, 42*, 1053–1067.

93. Safran, J. D., & Muran, J. C. (2000). *Negotiating the therapeutic alliance: A relational treatment guide.* New York: Guilford Press.

94. Gilbert, P., & Leahy, R. (Eds.). (2007). *The therapeutic relationship in the cognitive behavioural therapies.* London: Routledge.

95. Freeston, M., Thwaites, R., & Bennett-Levy, J. (in preparation). *Horses for courses: Designing, adapting and implementing self-practice/self-reflection programmes.*

96. Bennett-Levy, J., & Beedie, A. (2007). The ups and downs of cognitive therapy training: What happens to trainees' perception of their competence during a cognitive therapy training course? *Behavioural and Cognitive Psychotherapy, 35,* 61–75.

97. Beck, J. S. (2005). *Cognitive therapy for challenging problems.* New York: Guilford Press.

98. Bennett-Levy, J., & Padesky, C. A. (2014). Use it or lose it: Post-workshop reflection enhances learning and utilization of CBT skills. *Cognitive and Behavioral Practice, 21,* 12–19.

99. Barnard, P. J. (2004). Bridging between basic theory and clinical practice. *Behaviour Research and Therapy, 42,* 977–1000.

100. Barnard, P. J. (2009). Depression and attention to two kinds of meaning: A cognitive perspective. *Psychoanalytic Psychotherapy, 23,* 248–262.

101. McCraty, R., & Rees, R. A. (2009). The central role of the heart in generating and sustaining positive emotions. In S. Lopez & C. R. Snyder (Eds.), *Oxford handbook of positive psychology* (pp. 527–536). New York: Oxford University Press.

102. Michalak, J., Mischnat, J., & Teismann, T. (in press). Sitting posture makes a difference— Embodiment effects on depressive memory bias. *Clinical Psychology and Psychotherapy.*

103. Niedenthal, P. M. (2007). Embodying emotion. *Science, 316,* 1002–1005.

104. Nummenmaa, L., Glerean, E., Hari, R., & Hietanen, J. K. (2014). Bodily maps of emotions. *Proceedings of the National Academy of Sciences, 111,* 646–651.

Index